NURSING DATASOURCE 1997

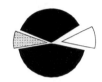

Volume I **Trends in Contemporary RN Nursing Education**

Pub. No. 19-7513

Center for Research in Nursing Education and Community Health

NATIONAL LEAGUE FOR NURSING

ISBN 0-88737-751-3

Printed in the United States of America.

PREFACE

Welcome to the comprehensive **Nursing DataSource 1997, Volume I**—a summation of findings from NLN's Annual Survey of Nursing Education Programs. Volume I, *Trends in Contemporary RN Nursing Education*, focuses on RN education programs. I am sure you will find the variety and depth of data and analysis presented in **Nursing DataSource 1997** a valuable resource for your own research needs. This volume is especially important for all of us to review and analyze carefully as we transform nursing education to match the changing face of health care.

The following Executive Summary highlights the trends that are emerging in this already changing system of care, explains the reasons for these trends, and anticipates what we can expect in the future. The pages of tables, graphs, and charts clearly expand upon this general analysis for further understanding and extrapolation of data.

NLN has continued to grow and expand to match a profession whose needs are many and whose future is invaluable to healthy communities. Indeed, please look over the following page to learn more about the **NLN Center for Research in Nursing Education and Community Health**. This Center maintains and enhances NLN's commitment to providing the essential information reported in **Nursing DataSource 1997, Volume I.**

Delroy Louden, PhD, FRSH
Executive Director
Center for Research in Nursing Education
    and Community Health
National League for Nursing

NLN CENTER FOR RESEARCH IN NURSING EDUCATION AND COMMUNITY HEALTH

The NLN Center for Research in Nursing Education and Community Health serves as a linking resource for nursing education and practice, research initiatives, community health care delivery, and information. For example, the Center serves as a repository of nursing education statistics and will maintain and expand NLN's national data bank, conduct research, and publish results of surveys and studies.

Since 1953, NLN Research has been maintaining and updating a comprehensive data bank on all state-approved nursing education programs. NLN's Annual Survey is conducted using a sophisticated research design and rigorous data collection methodology. Every year, with the cooperation of each state board of nursing, NLN Research surveys the more than 3,000 nursing education programs in operation within the United States.

The NLN Center for Research in Nursing Education and Community Health is also exploring new opportunities to create a dialogue with members of the research community. To accomplish this, the Center has initiated the following programs:

Seminars—NLN has brought together intimate groups of major thinkers to discuss contemporary issues and set direction for policy, planning, and implementation. NLN's First Annual Research Institute held in August, 1995 focused on community-based nursing and public health. In 1996, NLN Research continued the series with the Second Annual Research Institute on October 28-31, 1996 at NLN headquarters in New York City. The theme was "Measuring, Monitoring, and Evaluating the Health of Our Diverse Populations."

Training—NLN welcomes pre- and post-doctoral students from the fields of nursing, sociology, psychology, and epidemiology. In addition, faculty visit on an ongoing basis from around the world. In 1995, NLN welcomed two faculty members from Thailand who received training in research methodology. In 1996, faculty from South Africa, Spain and England also visited.

Internships—NLN offers internships to provide meaningful research experiences that will foster the development of the next generation of health researchers. The interns have access to NLN Research's database, or they may use data which they have collected, to provide them with hands-on experience in statistical analysis.

In addition, the Center has expanded into community-based research that is data driven and population-focused. Many of these special initiatives are collaborative, joining the Center with partners from new arenas ranging from small communities to sister organizations across the globe.

For further information about other publications and activities available through the NLN Center for Research in Nursing Education and Community Health, call 800-669-9656, ext. 166, or use our internet address: nlninform@nln.org.

Contents

Section 1
Executive Summary

EXECUTIVE SUMMARY

RESULTS FROM 1996 ANNUAL SURVEY

According to the results from the 1996 Annual Survey of RN programs, which was sent to all state-approved schools of nursing, declining trends were pervasive for the overall number of basic RN programs and students.

NUMBER OF PROGRAMS

For the first time since 1989, the overall number of basic RN programs declined, dropping from 1,516 in 1995 to 1,508 in 1996 (Figure 1). The reduction did not include baccalaureate programs which increased by two, but resulted from the loss of ten diploma programs. The number of associate degree programs remained constant (Figure 2).

ENROLLMENTS

Since 1994, overall enrollments have been declining, with a steep drop of 8.8 percent in 1996, from 261,219 students in 1995 to 238,244 students in 1996 (Figure 3). Enrollments declined across program type, with associate degree declining by 9.6 percent, diploma declining by 22.4 percent and basic baccalaureate declining by 5.7 percent (Figure 4).

The decline in enrollments was limited to basic students, i.e., students who did not have an RN license (Figure 5). Post-RN enrollments increased by 2 percent, from 47,100 in 1995 to 48,030 in 1996. The increase was limited to basic baccalaureate programs (programs that were state-approved to prepare for RN licensure), increasing by 5.2 percent (Figure 6). Post-RN enrollments in BRN programs (programs that offered a nursing program for RNs only) decreased by 2 percent, in contrast to 1995 where BRN enrollments increased by 20 percent. Possible reasons for the increased post-RN enrollments in basic baccalaureate, as compared to BRN programs, include an increased percentage of RNs attending school full-time, a schedule more typical in basic programs, and a higher percentage of basic programs which offered alternative schedules, particularly evening classes which increased from 58 percent to 65 percent between 1995 and 1996.

ANNUAL ADMISSIONS

For the second consecutive year overall annual admissions declined, going from 127,184 in 1995 to 119,205 in 1996, a decrease of 6.3 percent (Figure 7). Basic baccalaureate admissions declined for the first time since 1988, going from 43,451 in 1995 to 40,048 in 1996, a decrease of 7.8 percent.

Annual admissions to associate degree programs dropped by 4.1 percent, and diploma program admissions dropped by 19.3 percent.

GRADUATES

The decline in associate degree and diploma enrollments continued to impact the number of graduates from these programs, to the point where the overall number of graduates declined for the first time since 1990, declining by 2.4 percent (Figure 8). Between 1995 and 1996, associate degree graduates decreased by 3.6 percent, and diploma graduates decreased by 19.1 percent. While the number of basic baccalaureate graduates increased by 3.7 percent, it is anticipated that these programs will shortly see the impact of declining enrollments as well. The percentage of post-RN graduates also increased from both basic and BRN programs, 13.6 percent and 25.5 percent, respectively.

FALL ADMISSIONS

Fall admissions, which provide the number of first time students admitted into RN programs between August 1, 1996 through December 31, 1996, reflect the latest data on admission trends. Fall admissions have been declining since 1994, and this pattern continued, dropping from 88,901 in 1995, to 83,629 in 1996, a decline of 5.9 percent (Figure 9). These declines occurred across program type, with fall admissions from basic baccalaureate programs declining by 3.9 percent, associate degree programs declining by 5.7 percent, and diploma programs declining by 20.5 percent (Figure 10).

The application rate in relation to fall admissions provides a rough indication of demand for entry into nursing education. The overall number of applications per fall admission dropped from 2.75 in 1995 to 2.43 in 1996. This overall rate was representative of the declining rate across program type, which indicates a general decline in the application rate for basic nursing education.

ANNUAL TUITION

Tuition at publicly financed programs remained stable between 1995 and 1996, with tuition increasing for state residents by 0.8 percent, while decreasing for non-residents by 0.3 percent. However, tuition at private schools increased by 10.4 percent, going from $7,970 in 1995 to $8,801 in 1996. The highest average annual tuition was at private basic baccalaureate programs ($11,028), while the lowest was at public associate degree programs where state residents paid an average of $1,594 per year.

MINORITY ENROLLMENTS AND GRADUATES

In 1996 a higher percentage of minority students, approximately 20 percent, were admitted and enrolled in RN programs as compared to the previous year (Figure 11). However, there was an increasing disparity with black students between percent enrolled as compared to percent graduated (Figure 12). For example, during the early 1990's enrollment of black students consistently approximated 9 percent. However, during the mid 1990's the percentage of black students who graduated has consistently approximated 7 percent. This gap was more pronounced with black students, as compared to the other minority groups, and occurred across program type. Further study would be needed to determine if this pattern results from greater part-time rather than full-time enrollment, or it results from students not completing the programs.

4

ENROLLMENT OF MEN IN NURSING PROGRAMS

The percentage of men admitted and enrolled in RN programs declined slightly, going from approximately 13 percent in 1995 to 12 percent in 1996. The percentage of men who graduated remained constant at just over 12 percent. During the mid-1980s the percentage of men entering the nursing profession steadily increased, representing 4 percent of enrollments in 1986 and growing to 12 percent by 1993. However, since 1993 there have been nominal changes, with the percentage enrolled fluctuating between 12 and 13 percent. This seems to indicate that the number of men entering nursing has reached a plateau.

HISTORICAL PERSPECTIVE

In 1978 the Director of the NLN Division of Research, Dr. Walter Johnson, examined the history of growth in basic nursing education with respect to the number of programs and annual admissions.[1] Dr. Johnson described three phases of growth in nursing education, each lasting approximately ten years. Phase One, from 1948 to 1958, experienced very little growth. In Phase Two, from 1959 through 1967, admissions increased rapidly primarily due to the growth of associate degree programs. However, the greatest expansion occurred in Phase Three, which lasted from 1968 through 1977, with an increase in baccalaureate programs along with the continued growth of associate degree programs (Figure 13 and Figure 14). This expansion was the result of the shift in basic nursing education from hospital-based to college-based programs.[2]

In 1978, Dr. Johnson[1] suggested that nursing education was entering a fourth phase, "...one of retrenchment and cessation of growth. The PN programs stopped growing in 1970, and the aggregate admissions to RN programs have not grown significantly since 1974. This phase comprises the plateau nursing education has now entered." (p. 572).

Dr. Johnson's analysis can now be extended from 1978 to 1996. Phase Four (1978 through 1987) was initially characterized by a plateau, followed by several years of increases and then decreases. Phase Five, beginning in 1988, marked another period of great expansion. Annual admissions in basic nursing education programs experienced a seven-year growth period which peaked in 1994 with 129,897 students admitted. This growth came at a time when hospital demand for RNs increased with the implementation of the Prospective Payment System, and hospitals hired RNs, rather than LPNs or other patient care staff, to provide assessment and treatment to the increased level of acute care patients.[3] With increased demand came an increase in salary, growing from $17,398 in 1980 to 28,383 in 1988, an increase of 63 percent, and then to $37,738 in 1992, a 33 percent increase.[4,5]

However, with the advent of managed care and the subsequent cost constraints, a shift occurred with hospitals employing ancillary nursing personnel rather than RNs as a cost saving measure. As stated in the Institute of Medicine[3] report, "Labor costs account for a major proportion of hospital costs. When hospitals face pressures to cut costs, the usual target is labor. Increasing salary levels, combined with the increasing size of the RN workforce, have made RN employment a large and expensive cost center in the health care system" (p. 85).

The changing cycle was clearly evident in the results from the biennial NLN Newly Licensed Nurse Survey.[6,7] In the 1988 survey, 70 percent of new nurses reported "many jobs" were available to them, and in 1990, 63 percent reported this. However, in 1992 there was a noticeable shift with 37 percent of the new nurses reporting "many jobs" available and in the 1994 survey, the downward trend continued with only 6 percent reporting this.

The impact on nursing education was evident in the 1995 NLN Annual Survey when the question was asked whether the school planned to reduce admissions.[8] The percentage that planned reductions, according to program type, was: 59 percent of diploma programs; 26 percent of associate degree programs; 21 percent of basic baccalaureate programs; and 10 percent of BRN programs. The primary reasons given were lack of perceived job opportunities for the graduates, and reduced budgets.

At this point, basic nursing education seems to be in another period of retrenchment and cessation of growth, although post-RN education is expanding. While the hallmark of Phase Two and Phase Three was a shift in basic nursing education from *hospital* to *college-based* programs, the hallmark of Phase Six may be a shift from *basic* nursing education to *post-RN* education.

Donna Post, PhD
Director of Research
Center for Research in Nursing
Education & Community Health

Delroy Louden, PhD
Executive Director
Center for Research in Nursing
Education & Community Health

REFERENCES

1. Johnson, W.L. (1978). Educational preparation for nursing—1977. *Nursing Outlook, 26*(9), 568-573.

2. Dillon, P. (1997). The future of associate degree nursing. *N & HC Perspectives on Community, 18*(1), 20-24.

3. Wunderlich, G.S., Sloan, F.A., & Davis, C.K. (Eds.). (1996). *Nursing staff in hospitals and nursing homes: Is it adequate?* Washington, DC: National Academy Press.

4. Moses, E.B. (1990). *1988 The registered nurse population: Findings from the National Sample Survey of Registered Nurses, March 1988.* Washington, DC: Division of Nursing, Bureau of Health Professions, Health Resources and Services Administration.

5. Moses, E.B. (1994). *1992 The registered nurse population: Findings from the National Sample Survey of Registered Nurses, March 1992.* Washington, DC: Division of Nursing, Bureau of Health Professions, Health Resources and Services Administration.

6. Rosenfeld, P. (1994). *Profiles of the newly licensed nurse* (2nd ed.). New York: National League for Nursing Press.

7. Louden, D., Crawford, L., & Trotman, S. (1996). *Profiles of the newly licensed nurse* (3rd ed.). New York: National League for Nursing Press.

8. Post, D., & Louden, D. (1996). Executive summary. *Nursing DataSource 1996: Volume I-Trends in contemporary nursing education.* New York: National League for Nursing Press.

Section 2
Graphs

Figure 1
NUMBER OF BASIC RN PROGRAMS DECLINE

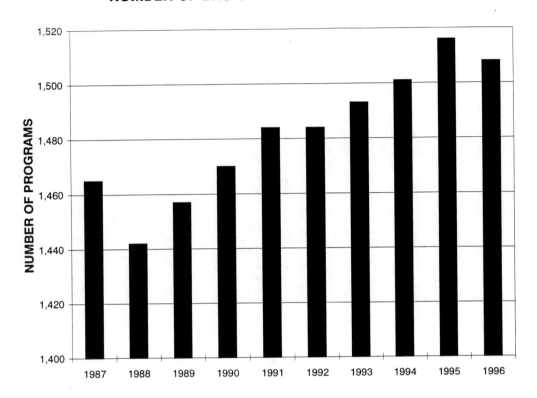

Figure 2
BASIC BACCALAUREATE PROGRAMS INCREASE IN NUMBER

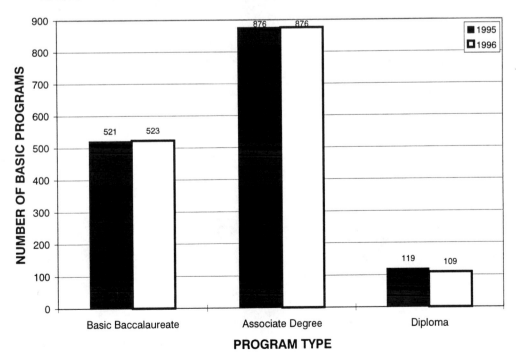

Figure 3
RN ENROLLMENTS CONTINUE TO DECLINE

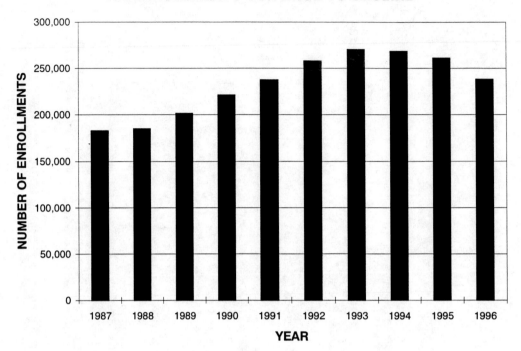

Figure 4
ENROLLMENTS DECLINE ACROSS PROGRAM TYPE

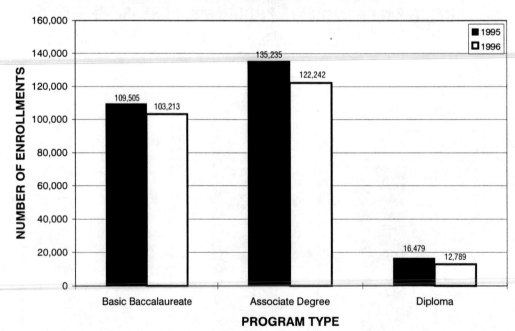

Figure 5
INCREASE IN POST-RN ENROLLMENTS

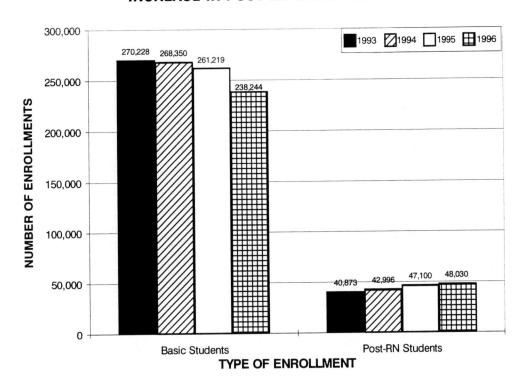

Figure 6
POST-RN ENROLLMENTS INCREASE IN BASIC PROGRAMS, BUT DECREASE IN BRN PROGRAMS

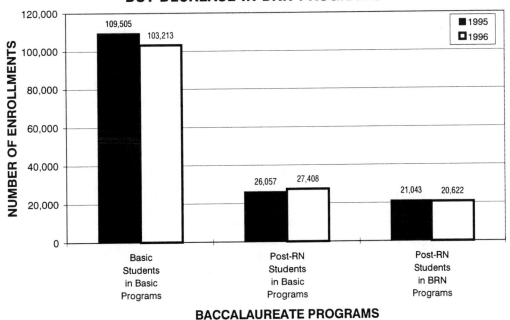

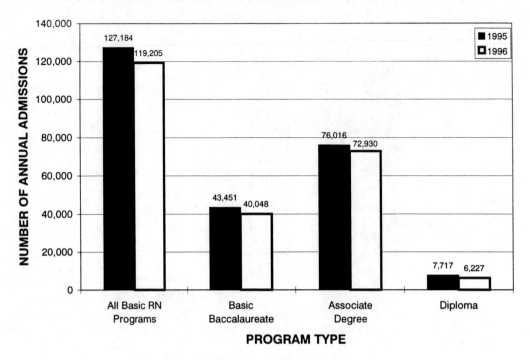

Figure 7
DECLINING ADMISSIONS OCCUR ACROSS PROGRAM TYPE

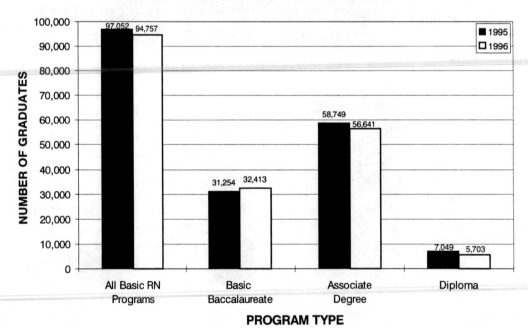

Figure 8
SOLE INCREASE WAS IN NUMBER OF
BASIC BACCALAUREATE GRADUATES

Figure 9
OVERALL FALL ADMISSIONS DECLINE FOR THIRD YEAR

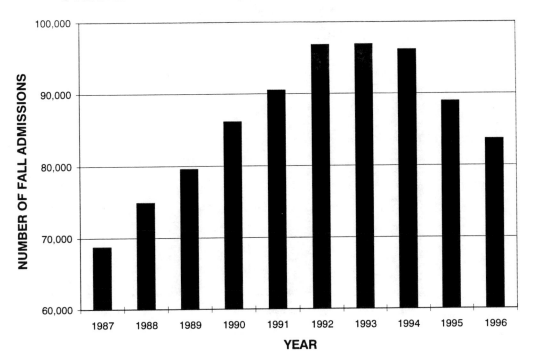

Figure 10
FALL ADMISSIONS DECLINE ACROSS PROGRAM TYPE

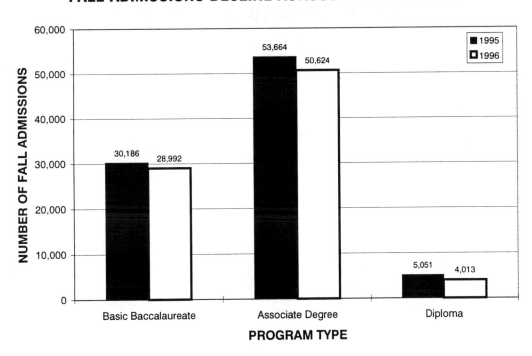

Figure 11
HIGHER PERCENTAGE OF MINORITY STUDENTS ENROLLED IN BASIC RN PROGRAMS

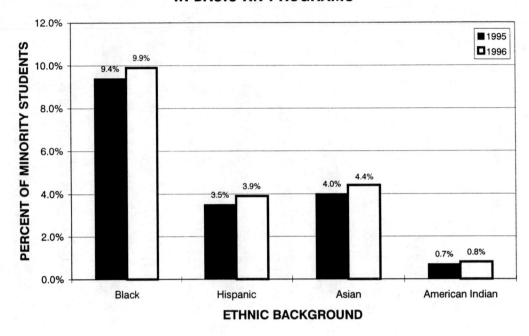

Figure 12
INCREASING DISPARITY BETWEEN PERCENTAGE OF BLACK STUDENTS ENROLLED VERSUS GRADUATED

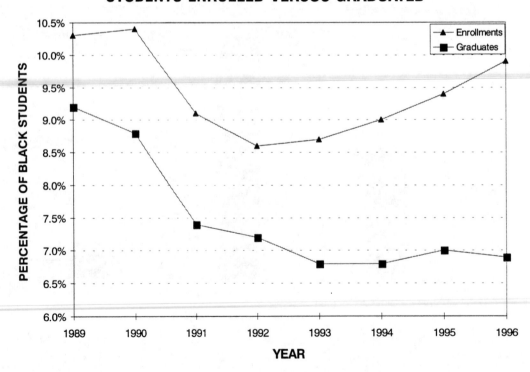

Figure 13
NUMBER OF BASIC RN PROGRAMS: 1958–1996

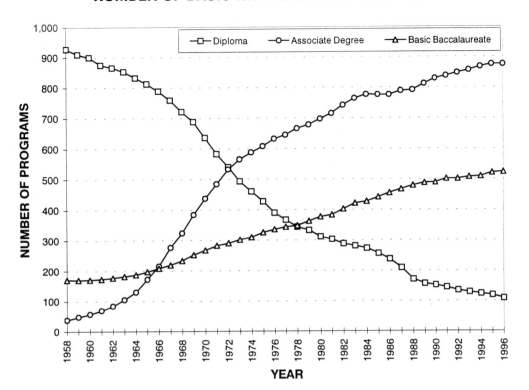

Figure 14
NUMBER OF ANNUAL ADMISSIONS TO
BASIC RN PROGRAMS: 1958–1996

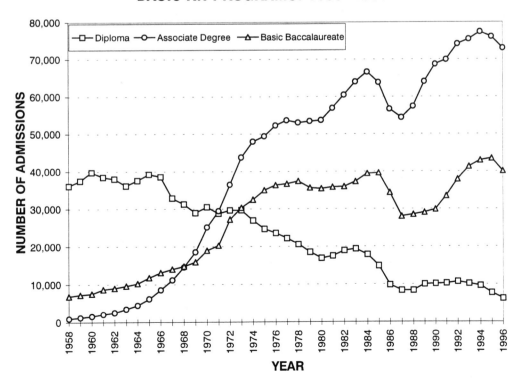

Section 3
Numeric Tables

Table 1
BASIC RN PROGRAMS AND PERCENTAGE CHANGE FROM PREVIOUS YEAR,
BY TYPE OF PROGRAM: 1976 TO 1996[1]

YEAR	NUMBER OF SCHOOLS	ALL BASIC RN PROGRAMS		BACCALAUREATE PROGRAMS		ASSOCIATE DEGREE PROGRAMS		DIPLOMA PROGRAMS	
		Number of Programs	Percent Change	Number of Programs	Percent Change	Number of Programs	Percent Change	Number of Programs	Percent Change
1976	1,337	1,358	-0.3	336	+3.1	632	+3.9	390	-8.9
1977	1,339	1,356	-0.1	344	+2.4	645	+2.1	367	-5.9
1978	1,340	1,358	+0.1	348	+1.2	666	+3.3	344	-6.3
1979	1,354	1,374	+1.2	363	+4.3	678	+1.8	333	-3.2
1980	1,360	1,385	+0.8	377	+3.9	697	+2.8	311	-6.6
1981	1,377	1,401	+1.2	383	+1.6	715	+2.6	303	-2.6
1982	1,406	1,432	+2.2	402	+5.0	742	+3.8	288	-5.0
1983	1,432	1,466	+2.4	421	+4.7	764	+3.0	281	-2.4
1984	1,445	1,477	+0.8	427	+1.4	777	+1.7	273	-2.8
1985	1,434	1,473	-0.2	441	+3.3	776	-0.1	256	-6.2
1986	1,426	1,469	-0.3	455	+3.2	776	-0.0	238	-7.0
1987	1,406	1,465	-0.3	467	+2.6	789	+1.7	209	-12.2
1988	1,391	1,442	-1.6	479	+2.6	792	+0.3	171	-18.7
1989	1,429	1,457	+1.0	488	+1.9	812	+2.5	157	-8.2
1990	1,412	1,470	+0.9	489	+0.2	829	+2.1	152	-3.2
1991	1,411	1,484	+1.0	501	+2.4	838	+1.1	145	-4.6
1992	1,404	1,484	+0.0	501	+0.0	848	+1.2	135	-6.9
1993	1,415[2]	1,493	+0.6	507	+1.2	857	+1.1	129	-4.4
1994	1,422	1,501	+0.5	509	+0.4	868	+1.3	124	-3.9
1995	1,434	1,516	+1.0	521	+2.4	876	+0.9	119	-4.0
1996	1,427	1,508	-0.5	523	+0.4	876	0.0	109	-8.4

[1] Excludes American Samoa, Guam, Puerto Rico, and the Virgin Islands.
[2] Updated information.

Table 2
PUBLIC AND PRIVATE BASIC RN PROGRAMS, BY TYPE OF PROGRAM: 1987 TO 1996[1]

PUBLIC AND PRIVATE NURSING PROGRAMS	NUMBER OF PROGRAMS									
	1987	1988	1989	1990	1991	1992	1993	1994	1995	1996
All Programs	1,465	1,442	1,457	1,470	1,484	1,484	1,493	1,501	1,516	1,508
Public	970	979	1,005	1,020	1.038	1,036	1,048	1,056	1,052	1,047
Private	495	463	452	450	446	448	445	445	464	461
Baccalaureate	467	479	488	489	501	501	507	509	521	523
Public	235	239	245	248	254	254	260	265	269	269
Private	232	240	243	241	247	247	247	244	252	254
Assoc. Degree	789	792	812	829	838	848	857	868	876	876
Public	698	704	726	741	750	754	758	764	766	764
Private	91	88	86	88	88	94	99	104	110	112
Diploma	209	171	157	152	145	135	129	124	119	109
Public	37	36	34	31	34	28	30	27	17	14
Private	172	135	123	121	111	107	99	97	102	95

[1] Excludes American Samoa, Guam, Puerto Rico, and the Virgin Islands.

Table 3
ALL BASIC RN PROGRAMS, BY NLN REGION AND STATE: 1987 TO 1996[1]

NLN REGION AND STATE	NUMBER OF PROGRAMS									
	1987	1988	1989	1990	1991	1992	1993	1994	1995	1996
United States	1,465	1,442	1,457	1,470	1,484	1,484	1,493	1,501	1,516	1,508
North Atlantic	355	343	335	331	335	332	329	329	331	327
Midwest	424	415	423	429	430	429	435	434	441	442
South	481	475	483	489	497	500	507	513	516	514
West	205	209	216	221	222	223	222	225	228	225
Alabama	35	35	35	34	33	34	34	36	36	36
Alaska	2	2	3	2	2	2	2	2	2	2
Arizona	15	15	15	15	15	16	16	16	17	17
Arkansas	21	21	21	21	23	24	24	22	22	22
California	89	90	91	91	92	93	93	94	96	95
Colorado	12	12	12	17	17	17	17	17	17	16
Connecticut	18	18	18	18	19	17	17	17	17	16
Delaware	6	6	7	7	7	7	7	7	7	7
D. of Columbia	6	5	5	5	5	5	5	5	5	5
Florida	40	40	40	39	39	40	40	40	40	39
Georgia	33	32	33	32	33	32	32	32	33	33
Hawaii	6	6	7	7	7	6	7	7	7	7
Idaho	7	7	7	7	7	7	7	7	8	7
Illinois	72	72	70	69	69	67	70	71	73	73
Indiana	40	42	44	46	44	46	46	46	46	46
Iowa	36	36	37	40	40	40	40	40	42	42
Kansas	32	33	32	32	32	30	30	30	30	29
Kentucky	27	27	29	32	32	33	34	34	35	34
Louisiana	22	21	21	23	23	21	22	23	23	23
Maine	15	15	14	14	14	14	15	15	15	15
Maryland	24	23	23	23	24	24	24	24	23	23
Massachusetts	48	44	41	42	43	42	42	43	44	44
Michigan	49	48	49	50	50	49	50	50	49	48
Minnesota	23	23	20	20	21	21	21	21	21	24
Mississippi	21	21	21	21	21	21	23	23	23	23
Missouri	42	40	44	45	47	46	47	46	48	50
Montana	4	4	5	5	5	5	5	5	5	5
Nebraska	13	10	13	15	13	13	13	13	14	14
Nevada	7	7	6	6	6	6	6	6	6	6
New Hampshire	10	10	9	9	9	9	9	9	9	9
New Jersey	38	38	38	39	38	38	37	37	38	37
New Mexico	13	14	14	14	14	14	14	16	15	15
New York	108	103	101	99	101	103	100	100	100	101
North Carolina	57	57	59	61	62	62	62	62	62	62
North Dakota	8	6	7	6	7	7	7	7	7	7
Ohio	70	67	68	67	68	69	70	69	69	67
Oklahoma	27	27	27	27	27	27	28	28	28	28
Oregon	17	18	18	18	18	18	16	16	16	16
Pennsylvania	94	92	90	87	88	86	86	84	84	82
Rhode Island	7	7	7	6	6	6	6	7	7	7
South Carolina	20	20	20	20	21	20	20	20	21	21
South Dakota	9	9	10	9	8	10	10	10	10	10
Tennessee	35	35	34	35	35	35	35	36	36	36
Texas	64	64	68	69	70	72	73	77	77	77
Utah	4	4	7	7	7	7	7	7	7	7
Vermont	5	5	5	5	5	5	5	5	5	4
Virginia	35	34	34	34	35	36	37	37	37	37
Washington	23	24	24	24	24	24	24	24	24	24
West Virginia	20	18	18	18	19	19	19	19	20	20
Wisconsin	30	29	29	30	31	31	31	31	32	32
Wyoming	6	6	7	8	8	8	8	8	8	8
American Samoa	1	1	1	1	1	1	1	1	1	1
Guam	1	1	1	1	1	1	1	1	1	1
Puerto Rico	20	22	22	22	25	28	29	31	31	37
Virgin Islands	2	2	2	2	2	2	2	2	2	2

[1] National and regional totals exclude American Samoa, Guam, Puerto Rico, and the Virgin Islands.

20

Table 4
BASIC BACCALAUREATE NURSING PROGRAMS, BY NLN REGION AND STATE: 1987 TO 1996[1]

NLN REGION AND STATE	NUMBER OF PROGRAMS									
	1987	1988	1989	1990	1991	1992	1993	1994	1995	1996
United States	467	479	488	489	501	501	507	509	521	523
North Atlantic	110	111	110	109	111	111	113	113	115	117
Midwest	144	151	157	157	161	159	161	160	164	164
South	158	162	165	165	170	172	175	177	181	181
West	55	55	56	58	59	59	58	59	61	61
Alabama	13	13	13	12	12	12	12	12	13	13
Alaska	1	1	1	1	1	1	1	1	1	1
Arizona	4	4	4	4	4	4	4	4	4	4
Arkansas	7	7	7	7	7	8	9	9	9	9
California	21	21	21	22	23	23	23	23	24	24
Colorado	6	6	6	7	7	7	7	7	7	7
Connecticut	7	7	7	7	7	7	8	8	8	8
Delaware	2	2	2	2	2	2	2	2	2	2
D. of Columbia	5	4	4	4	4	4	4	4	4	4
Florida	13	13	13	13	13	13	13	13	13	13
Georgia	12	12	13	12	12	12	12	12	13	14
Hawaii	2	2	2	2	2	2	3	3	3	3
Idaho	2	2	2	2	2	2	2	2	3	3
Illinois	24	26	27	27	28	27	27	27	27	27
Indiana	17	20	21	21	21	21	21	20	20	20
Iowa	11	11	11	12	12	12	12	12	12	12
Kansas	11	11	10	10	10	10	11	11	11	11
Kentucky	9	9	10	10	10	10	10	10	10	10
Louisiana	12	12	12	12	12	12	13	13	13	13
Maine	5	6	6	6	6	6	7	7	7	7
Maryland	6	6	6	6	7	7	7	7	7	7
Massachusetts	15	14	14	14	15	15	15	15	16	16
Michigan	14	14	14	14	14	13	14	14	15	15
Minnesota	11	11	8	8	9	9	9	9	9	9
Mississippi	7	7	7	7	7	7	7	7	7	7
Missouri	11	11	14	14	15	15	15	15	17	17
Montana	2	2	2	2	2	2	2	2	2	2
Nebraska	7	7	7	7	6	6	6	6	6	6
Nevada	2	2	2	2	2	2	2	2	2	2
New Hampshire	3	3	3	3	3	3	3	3	3	3
New Jersey	7	7	7	7	7	7	7	7	8	9
New Mexico	1	1	1	1	1	1	1	2	2	2
New York	32	33	32	31	32	32	32	32	32	33
North Carolina	12	12	12	12	12	12	12	12	12	12
North Dakota	4	6	7	6	7	7	7	7	7	7
Ohio	18	18	21	21	22	22	22	22	22	22
Oklahoma	11	11	11	11	11	11	11	11	11	11
Oregon	4	4	5	5	5	5	3	3	3	3
Pennsylvania	30	31	31	31	31	31	31	31	31	31
Rhode Island	3	3	3	3	3	3	3	3	3	3
South Carolina	6	7	7	7	7	7	7	7	8	8
South Dakota	3	3	4	4	4	4	4	4	4	4
Tennessee	12	14	14	15	16	16	16	17	18	18
Texas	20	21	22	23	24	25	25	26	26	25
Utah	3	3	3	3	3	3	3	3	3	3
Vermont	1	1	1	1	1	1	1	1	1	1
Virginia	10	10	10	10	11	11	12	12	12	12
Washington	6	6	6	6	6	6	6	6	6	6
West Virginia	8	8	8	8	9	9	9	9	9	9
Wisconsin	13	13	13	13	13	13	13	13	14	14
Wyoming	1	1	1	1	1	1	1	1	1	1
American Samoa	0	0	0	0	0	0	0	0	0	0
Guam	0	1	1	1	1	1	1	1	1	1
Puerto Rico	12	13	13	13	13	13	14	14	14	17
Virgin Islands	1	1	1	1	1	1	1	1	1	1

[1] National and regional totals exclude American Samoa, Guam, Puerto Rico, and the Virgin Islands.

Table 5
ASSOCIATE DEGREE NURSING PROGRAMS, BY NLN REGION AND STATE: 1986 TO 1995[1]

NLN REGION AND STATE	NUMBER OF PROGRAMS									
	1987	1988	1989	1990	1991	1992	1993	1994	1995	1996
United States	789	792	812	829	838	848	857	868	876	876
North Atlantic	147	146	148	147	151	152	151	153	153	152
Midwest	209	211	218	227	228	232	238	241	246	250
South	284	282	287	293	297	301	305	309	311	310
West	149	153	159	162	162	163	163	165	166	164
Alabama	20	20	20	20	20	21	21	23	23	23
Alaska	1	1	2	1	1	1	1	1	1	1
Arizona	11	11	11	11	11	12	12	12	13	13
Arkansas	12	12	12	12	14	14	13	11	11	11
California	67	68	69	68	68	69	69	70	71	71
Colorado	6	6	6	10	10	10	10	10	10	9
Connecticut	6	6	6	6	7	7	6	6	6	6
Delaware	3	3	4	4	4	4	4	4	4	4
D. of Columbia	1	1	4	1	1	1	1	1	1	1
Florida	26	26	26	25	25	26	26	26	26	26
Georgia	19	19	19	19	20	20	20	20	20	19
Hawaii	4	4	5	5	5	4	4	4	4	4
Idaho	5	5	5	5	5	5	5	5	5	4
Illinois	34	35	35	35	35	35	38	39	42	42
Indiana	17	19	20	23	22	24	24	25	25	25
Iowa	20	20	21	23	23	23	23	23	25	25
Kansas	19	20	21	21	21	19	19	19	19	18
Kentucky	18	18	19	22	22	23	24	24	25	24
Louisiana	6	6	6	8	8	8	8	9	9	9
Maine	9	9	8	8	8	8	8	8	8	8
Maryland	14	14	14	14	14	14	14	14	14	14
Massachusetts	20	19	19	20	20	20	20	21	21	21
Michigan	32	31	32	33	33	33	33	33	32	31
Minnesota	12	12	12	12	12	12	12	12	12	15
Mississippi	14	14	14	14	14	14	16	16	16	16
Missouri	22	21	22	23	24	25	26	27	27	30
Montana	2	2	3	3	3	3	3	3	3	3
Nebraska	1	2	5	7	6	6	6	6	7	7
Nevada	5	5	4	4	4	4	4	4	4	4
New Hampshire	6	6	6	6	6	6	6	6	6	6
New Jersey	14	14	14	15	14	14	14	14	14	14
New Mexico	12	13	13	13	13	13	13	14	13	13
New York	60	59	60	59	61	63	63	63	63	63
North Carolina	41	41	43	45	46	46	46	46	47	47
North Dakota	2	0	0	0	0	0	0	0	0	0
Ohio	30	31	30	30	31	32	34	34	34	34
Oklahoma	16	16	16	16	16	16	17	17	17	17
Oregon	13	14	13	13	13	13	13	13	13	13
Pennsylvania	22	23	24	22	24	23	23	23	23	23
Rhode Island	2	2	2	2	2	2	2	3	3	3
South Carolina	13	13	13	13	14	13	13	13	13	13
South Dakota	5	5	5	4	4	6	6	6	6	6
Tennessee	17	17	16	16	15	15	15	15	14	14
Texas	42	41	44	44	44	45	46	49	49	50
Utah	1	1	4	4	4	4	4	4	4	4
Vermont	4	4	4	4	4	4	4	4	4	3
Virginia	16	16	16	16	16	17	17	17	17	17
Washington	17	18	18	18	18	18	18	18	18	18
West Virginia	10	9	9	9	9	9	9	9	10	10
Wisconsin	15	15	15	16	17	17	17	17	17	17
Wyoming	5	5	6	7	7	7	7	7	7	7
American Samoa	1	1	1	1	1	1	1	1	1	1
Guam	1	0	0	0	0	0	0	0	0	0
Puerto Rico	8	9	9	9	12	15	15	17	17	20
Virgin Islands	1	1	1	1	1	1	1	1	1	1

[1] National and regional totals exclude American Samoa, Guam, Puerto Rico, and the Virgin Islands.

Table 6
DIPLOMA NURSING PROGRAMS, BY NLN REGION AND STATE: 1987 TO 1996[1]

NLN REGION AND STATE	NUMBER OF PROGRAMS									
	1987	1988	1989	1990	1991	1992	1993	1994	1995	1996
United States	209	171	157	152	145	135	129	124	119	109
North Atlantic	98	86	77	75	73	69	65	63	63	58
Midwest	71	53	48	45	41	38	36	33	31	28
South	39	31	31	31	30	27	27	27	24	23
West	1	1	1	1	1	1	1	1	1	0
Alabama	2	2	2	2	1	1	1	1	0	0
Alaska	0	0	0	0	0	0	0	0	0	0
Arizona	0	0	0	0	0	0	0	0	0	0
Arkansas	2	2	2	2	2	2	2	2	2	2
California	1	1	1	1	1	1	1	1	1	0
Colorado	0	0	0	0	0	0	0	0	0	0
Connecticut	5	5	5	5	5	3	3	3	3	2
Delaware	1	1	1	1	1	1	1	1	1	1
D. of Columbia	0	0	0	0	0	0	0	0	0	0
Florida	1	1	1	1	1	1	1	1	1	0
Georgia	2	1	1	1	1	0	0	0	0	0
Hawaii	0	0	0	0	0	0	0	0	0	0
Idaho	0	0	0	0	0	0	0	0	0	0
Illinois	14	11	8	7	6	5	5	5	4	4
Indiana	6	3	3	2	1	1	1	1	1	1
Iowa	5	5	5	5	5	5	5	5	5	5
Kansas	2	2	1	1	1	1	0	0	0	0
Kentucky	0	0	0	0	0	0	0	0	0	0
Louisiana	4	3	3	3	3	1	1	1	1	1
Maine	1	0	0	0	0	0	0	0	0	0
Maryland	4	3	3	3	3	3	3	3	2	2
Massachusetts	13	11	8	8	8	7	7	7	7	7
Michigan	3	3	3	3	3	3	3	3	2	2
Minnesota	0	0	0	0	0	0	0	0	0	0
Mississippi	0	0	0	0	0	0	0	0	0	0
Missouri	9	8	8	8	8	6	6	4	4	3
Montana	0	0	0	0	0	0	0	0	0	0
Nebraska	5	1	1	1	1	1	1	1	1	1
Nevada	0	0	0	0	0	0	0	0	0	0
New Hampshire	1	1	0	0	0	0	0	0	0	0
New Jersey	17	17	17	17	17	17	16	16	16	14
New Mexico	0	0	0	0	0	0	0	0	0	0
New York	16	11	9	9	8	8	5	5	5	5
North Carolina	4	4	4	4	4	4	4	4	3	3
North Dakota	2	0	0	0	0	0	0	0	0	0
Ohio	22	18	17	16	15	15	14	13	13	11
Oklahoma	0	0	0	0	0	0	0	0	0	0
Oregon	0	0	0	0	0	0	0	0	0	0
Pennsylvania	42	38	35	34	33	32	32	30	30	28
Rhode Island	2	2	2	1	1	1	1	1	1	1
South Carolina	1	0	0	0	0	0	0	0	0	0
South Dakota	1	1	1	1	0	0	0	0	0	0
Tennessee	6	4	4	4	4	4	4	4	4	4
Texas	2	2	2	2	2	2	2	2	2	2
Utah	0	0	0	0	0	0	0	0	0	0
Vermont	0	0	0	0	0	0	0	0	0	0
Virginia	9	8	8	8	8	8	8	8	8	8
Washington	0	0	0	0	0	0	0	0	0	0
West Virginia	2	1	1	1	1	1	1	1	1	1
Wisconsin	2	1	1	1	1	1	1	1	1	1
Wyoming	0	0	0	0	0	0	0	0	0	0
American Samoa	0	0	0	0	0	0	0	0	0	0
Guam	0	0	0	0	0	0	0	0	0	0
Puerto Rico	0	0	0	0	0	0	0	0	0	0
Virgin Islands	0	0	0	0	0	0	0	0	0	0

[1] National and regional totals exclude American Samoa, Guam, Puerto Rico, and the Virgin Islands.

Table 7
BACCALAUREATE NURSING PROGRAMS THAT ENROLL BASIC AND/OR RN STUDENTS,
BY NLN ACCREDITATION STATUS: JANUARY, 1997*

NLN ACCREDITATION STATUS	TOTAL NUMBER OF PROGRAMS	TYPE OF STUDENT ENROLLED	
		Both Basic and RN Students	RN Students Only
Total	672	523	149
Accredited	634	506	128
Non-Accredited	38	17	21

*Excludes American Samoa, Guam, Puerto Rico, and the Virgin Islands.

24

Table 8a
BASIC RN PROGRAMS BY NLN ACCREDITATION STATUS,
REGION AND STATE: JANUARY, 1997*

NLN REGION AND STATE	Total	Accredited	Not Accredited
United States	1,508	1,237	271
North Atlantic	327	300	27
Midwest	442	350	92
South	514	426	88
West	225	161	64
Alabama	36	32	4
Alaska	2	2	0
Arizona	17	14	3
Arkansas	22	20	2
California	95	52	43
Colorado	16	10	6
Connecticut	16	16	0
Delaware	7	6	1
D. of Columbia	5	5	0
Florida	39	30	9
Georgia	33	32	1
Hawaii	7	5	2
Idaho	7	7	0
Illinois	73	54	19
Indiana	46	41	5
Iowa	42	24	18
Kansas	29	28	1
Kentucky	34	26	8
Louisiana	23	22	1
Maine	15	15	0
Maryland	23	18	5
Massachusetts	44	42	2
Michigan	48	27	21
Minnesota	24	17	7
Mississippi	23	21	2
Missouri	50	36	14
Montana	5	5	0
Nebraska	14	13	1
Nevada	6	6	0
New Hampshire	9	7	2
New Jersey	37	36	1
New Mexico	15	12	3
New York	101	82	19
North Carolina	62	24	38
North Dakota	7	7	0
Ohio	67	64	3
Oklahoma	28	28	0
Oregon	16	11	5
Pennsylvania	82	81	1
Rhode Island	7	6	1
South Carolina	21	17	4
South Dakota	10	8	2
Tennessee	36	34	2
Texas	77	66	11
Utah	7	7	0
Vermont	4	4	0
Virginia	37	37	0
Washington	24	22	2
West Virginia	20	19	1
Wisconsin	32	31	1
Wyoming	8	8	0
American Samoa	1	0	1
Guam	1	1	0
Puerto Rico	37	12	25
Virgin Islands	2	2	0

*National and regional totals exclude American Samoa, Guam, Puerto Rico, and the Virgin Islands.

Table 8b
BASIC RN PROGRAMS, BY TYPE OF PROGRAM AND NLN ACCREDITATION STATUS: JANUARY, 1997*

NLN REGION AND STATE	NUMBER OF PROGRAMS							
	BACCALAUREATE PROGRAMS			ASSOCIATE DEGREE PROGRAMS			DIPLOMA PROGRAMS**	
	Total	Accredited	Not Accredited	Total	Accredited	Not Accredited	Total	Accredited
United States	523	506	17	876	622	254	109	109
North Atlantic	117	115	2	152	127	25	58	58
Midwest	164	159	5	250	163	87	28	28
South	181	172	9	310	231	79	23	23
West	61	60	1	164	101	63	0	0
Alabama	13	12	1	23	20	3	0	0
Alaska	1	1	0	1	1	0	0	0
Arizona	4	4	0	13	10	3	0	0
Arkansas	9	8	1	11	10	1	2	2
California	24	24	0	71	28	43	0	0
Colorado	7	7	0	9	3	6	0	0
Connecticut	8	8	0	6	6	0	2	2
Delaware	2	2	0	4	3	1	1	1
D. of Columbia	4	4	0	1	1	0	0	0
Florida	13	12	1	26	18	8	0	0
Georgia	14	13	1	19	19	0	0	0
Hawaii	3	2	1	4	3	1	0	0
Idaho	3	3	0	4	4	0	0	0
Illinois	27	25	2	42	25	17	4	4
Indiana	20	20	0	25	20	5	1	1
Iowa	12	12	0	25	7	18	5	5
Kansas	11	11	0	18	17	1	0	0
Kentucky	10	10	0	24	16	8	0	0
Louisiana	13	13	0	9	8	1	1	1
Maine	7	7	0	8	8	0	0	0
Maryland	7	7	0	14	9	5	2	2
Massachusetts	16	16	0	21	19	2	7	7
Michigan	15	14	1	31	11	20	2	2
Minnesota	9	9	0	15	8	7	0	0
Mississippi	7	7	0	16	14	2	0	0
Missouri	17	16	1	30	17	13	3	3
Montana	2	2	0	3	3	0	0	0
Nebraska	6	6	0	7	6	1	1	1
Nevada	2	2	0	4	4	0	0	0
New Hampshire	3	3	0	6	4	2	0	0
New Jersey	9	8	1	14	14	0	14	14
New Mexico	2	2	0	13	10	3	0	0
New York	33	32	1	63	45	18	5	5
North Carolina	12	12	0	47	9	38	3	3
North Dakota	7	7	0	0	0	0	0	0
Ohio	22	22	0	34	31	3	11	11
Oklahoma	11	11	0	17	17	0	0	0
Oregon	3	3	0	13	8	5	0	0
Pennsylvania	31	31	0	23	22	1	28	28
Rhode Island	3	3	0	3	2	1	1	1
South Carolina	8	6	2	13	11	2	0	0
South Dakota	4	4	0	6	4	2	0	0
Tennessee	18	16	2	14	14	0	4	4
Texas	25	24	1	50	40	10	2	2
Utah	3	3	0	4	4	0	0	0
Vermont	1	1	0	3	3	0	0	0
Virginia	12	12	0	17	17	0	8	8
Washington	6	6	0	18	16	2	0	0
West Virginia	9	9	0	10	9	1	1	1
Wisconsin	14	13	1	17	17	0	1	1
Wyoming	1	1	0	7	7	0	0	0
American Samoa	0	0	0	1	0	1	0	0
Guam	1	1	0	0	0	0	0	0
Puerto Rico	17	7	10	20	5	15	0	0
Virgin Islands	1	1	0	1	1	0	0	0

*National and regional totals exclude American Samoa, Guam, Puerto Rico, and the Virgin Islands.
**All Diploma programs were accredited.

Table 9
MEAN ANNUAL TUITIONS OF FULL-TIME STUDENTS IN PUBLIC OR PRIVATE
BASIC RN PROGRAMS: 1996 TO 1997[1]

| NURSING PROGRAMS | PRINCIPAL FINANCIAL SUPPORT OF SCHOOL | | |
| | Public | | Private |
	Resident	Non-Resident	
All Programs	$2,000	$4,956	$8,801
Basic Baccalaureate	$2,850	$7,099	$11,028
Associate Degree	$1,594	$4,104	$7,064
Diploma	$4,794	$5,828	$4,614

[1]Excludes American Samoa, Guam, Puerto Rico,
and the Virgin Islands.

Table 10
FALL ADMISSIONS TO PUBLIC AND PRIVATE BASIC RN PROGRAMS, BY TYPE OF PROGRAM: 1987 TO 1996[1]

| PUBLIC AND PRIVATE NURSING PROGRAMS | NUMBER OF FALL ADMISSIONS | | | | | | | | | |
	1987	1988	1989	1990	1991	1992	1993	1994	1995	1996
All Programs	68,745	74,921	79,570	86,125	90,499	96,786	96,864	96,107	88,901	83,629
Public	51,362	56,922	60,032	64,410	67,163	70,106	70,216	69,761	64,815	61,623
Private	17,383	17,999	19,538	21,715	23,336	26,680	26,648	26,346	24,086	22,006
Baccalaureate	19,985	20,749	21,544	25,117	27,361	31,719	32,403	33,124	30,186	28,992
Public	12,806	13,122	13,574	15,648	16,369	18,064	18,542	18,422	17,388	16,600
Private	7,179	7,627	7,970	9,469	10,992	13,655	13,861	14,702	12,798	12,392
Assoc. Degree	41,695	46,910	49,930	52,674	54,732	56,828	56,514	56,035	53,664	50,624
Public	37,389	42,357	44,840	47,175	49,124	50,777	50,170	50,200	46,998	44,584
Private	4,306	4,553	5,090	5,499	5,608	6,051	6,344	5,835	6,666	6,040
Diploma	7,065	7,262	8,096	8,334	8,406	8,239	7,947	6,948	5,051	4,013
Public	1,167	1,443	1,618	1,587	1,670	1,265	1,504	1,139	429	439
Private	5,898	5,819	6,478	6,747	6,736	6,974	6,443	5,809	4,622	3,574

[1] Excludes American Samoa, Guam, Puerto Rico, and the Virgin Islands.

Table 11
ANNUAL ADMISSIONS TO BASIC RN PROGRAMS AND PERCENTAGE CHANGE
FROM PREVIOUS YEAR, BY TYPE OF PROGRAM: 1976-77 TO 1995-96[1]

ACADEMIC YEAR	ALL BASIC RN PROGRAMS		BACCALAUREATE PROGRAMS		ASSOCIATE DEGREE PROGRAMS		DIPLOMA PROGRAMS	
	Number of Admissions	Percent Change	Number of Admissions	Percent Change	Number of Admissions	Percent Change	Number of Admissions	Percent Change
1976-77	112,523	+0.3	36,670	+1.0	53,610	+2.6	22,243	-5.8
1977-78	110,950	-1.4	37,348	+1.8	52,991	-1.1	20,611	-7.3
1978-79	107,476	-3.2	35,611	-4.7	53,366	+0.7	18,499	-10.2
1979-80	105,952	-1.4	35,414	-0.5	53,633	+0.5	16,905	-8.6
1980-81	110,201	+4.0	35,808	+1.1	56,899	+6.1	17,494	+3.5
1981-82	115,279	+4.6	35,928	+0.3	60,423	+6.1	18,928	+8.1
1982-83	120,579	+4.6	37,264	+3.7	63,947	+5.8	19,368	+2.3
1983-84	123,824	+2.7	39,400	+5.7	66,576	+4.1	17,848	-7.8
1984-85	118,224	-4.5	39,573	+0.4	63,776	-4.2	14,875	-16.7
1985-86	100,791	-14.7	34,310	-13.3	56,635	-11.2	9,846	-33.0
1986-87	90,693	-10.0	28,026	-18.3	54,330	-4.1	8,337	-15.3
1987-88	94,269	+3.9	28,505	+1.7	57,375	+5.6	8,389	+0.6
1988-89	103,025	+9.3	29,042	+1.9	63,973	+11.5	10,010	+19.3
1989-90	108,580	+5.4	29,858	+2.6	68,634	+7.3	10,088	+0.8
1990-91	113,526	+4.6	33,437	+12.0	69,869	+1.8	10,220	-1.3
1991-92	122,656	+8.0	37,886	+13.3	74,079	+6.0	10,691	+4.6
1992-93	126,837	+3.4	41,290	+9.0	75,382	+1.7	10,165	-4.9
1993-94	129,897	+2.4	42,953	+4.0	77,343	+2.6	9,601	-5.5
1994-95	127,184	-2.1	43,451	+1.2	76,016	-1.7	7,717	-19.6
1995-96	119,205	-6.3	40,048	-7.8	72,930	-4.1	6,227	-19.3

[1] Excludes American Samoa, Guam, Puerto Rico, and the Virgin Islands.

Table 12
ANNUAL ADMISSIONS TO PUBLIC AND PRIVATE BASIC RN PROGRAMS, BY TYPE OF PROGRAM: 1986-87 TO 1995-96[1]

PUBLIC AND PRIVATE NURSING PROGRAMS	NUMBER OF ANNUAL ADMISSIONS									
	1986-87	1987-88	1988-89	1989-90	1990-91	1991-92	1992-93	1993-94	1994-95	1995-96
All Programs	90,693	94,269	103,025	108,580	113,526	122,656	126,837	129,897	127,184	119,205
Public	67,890	71,866	77,892	82,686	88,764	92,720	94,572	96,296	89,819	86,917
Private	22,803	22,403	25,133	25,894	24,762	29,936	32,265	33,601	37,365	32,288
Baccalaureate	28,026	28,505	29,042	29,858	33,437	37,886	41,290	42,953	43,451	40,048
Public	18,057	18,622	18,824	19,492	22,252	23,484	24,345	24,861	24,909	23,262
Private	9,969	9,883	10,218	10,366	11,185	14,402	16,945	18,092	18,542	16,786
Assoc. Degree	54,330	57,375	63,973	68,634	69,869	74,079	75,382	77,343	76,016	72,930
Public	48,249	51,566	56,958	61,151	64,258	67,146	68,075	69,562	64,012	63,049
Private	6,081	5,809	7,015	7,483	5,611	6,933	7,307	7,781	12,004	9,881
Diploma	8,337	8,389	10,010	10,088	10,220	10,691	10,165	9,601	7,717	6,227
Public	1,584	1,678	2,110	2,043	2,254	2,090	2,152	1,873	898	606
Private	6,753	6,711	7,900	8,045	7,966	8,601	8,013	7,728	6,819	5,621

[1] Excludes American Samoa, Guam, Puerto Rico, and the Virgin Islands.

28

Table 13
ANNUAL ADMISSIONS TO ALL BASIC RN PROGRAMS, BY NLN REGION AND STATE: 1986-87 TO 1995-96[1]

NLN REGION AND STATE	NUMBER OF ADMISSIONS									
	1986-87	1987-88	1988-89	1989-90	1990-91	1991-92	1992-93	1993-94	1994-95	1995-96
United States	90,693	94,269	103,025	108,580	113,526	122,656	126,837	129,897	127,184	119,205
North Atlantic	23,069	23,792	25,876	26,889	27,349	30,556	32,589	33,140	32,757	29,600
Midwest	25,151	24,647	26,862	28,410	29,602	32,527	33,579	34,840	34,225	32,060
South	29,632	32,380	36,083	39,397	42,468	45,062	45,764	46,979	45,311	42,945
West	12,841	13,450	14,204	13,884	14,107	14,511	14,905	14,938	14,891	14,600
Alabama	2,149	2,003	2,346	2,574	2,570	3,108	3,488	3,847	3,718	3,438
Alaska	166	166	266	81	103	102	105	110	108	111
Arizona	962	970	996	929	1,110	1,196	1,237	1,281	1,369	1,415
Arkansas	983	1,327	1,415	1,545	1,723	1,821	1,802	1,751	1,500	1,398
California	6,098	6,320	6,507	6,340	6,465	6,577	6,691	6,710	6,998	6,814
Colorado	942	873	1,092	926	1,011	1,020	1,064	1,041	1,098	931
Connecticut	1,012	1,200	1,200	1,070	1,141	1,513	1,370	1,049	1,291	1,095
Delaware	339	370	386	394	316	455	580	532	561	422
D. of Columbia	334	449	315	248	361	327	555	355	373	335
Florida	3,426	3,651	3,849	4,400	4,551	4,688	4,930	4,835	5,173	5,094
Georgia	1,805	2,075	2,289	2,725	2,566	3,003	3,252	3,366	3,298	2,890
Hawaii	183	345	272	361	281	301	409	395	337	381
Idaho	274	391	332	338	372	331	333	352	330	341
Illinois	4,422	3,840	4,642	4,453	4,889	5,284	5,317	5,774	6,316	5,852
Indiana	2,480	2,496	2,581	2,594	2,820	3,038	3,213	3,257	3,404	3,595
Iowa	1,661	1,668	1,672	1,852	1,938	2,146	2,418	2,358	2,279	2,087
Kansas	957	1,165	1,244	1,613	1,521	1,610	1,831	1,603	1,565	1,426
Kentucky	1,683	1,879	2,093	2,159	3,048	2,729	2,676	2,757	2,596	2,421
Louisiana	1,432	1,558	1,741	2,081	3,100	2,970	2,813	3,156	2,984	2,193
Maine	433	421	514	498	579	490	797	602	820	655
Maryland	1,483	1,449	1,542	1,566	1,819	2,166	2,268	2,269	2,070	2,138
Massachusetts	2,700	2,545	2,536	3,082	3,020	3,415	3,422	3,386	3,277	3,337
Michigan	3,872	3,521	3,582	3,748	3,890	4,308	4,139	4,236	4,120	3,943
Minnesota	1,431	1,570	1,788	1,939	1,759	1,974	2,042	1,997	1,915	1,882
Mississippi	1,503	1,440	1,584	1,988	2,089	2,144	2,184	2,211	2,117	2,155
Missouri	2,087	1,962	2,196	2,350	2,535	3,049	2,999	3,380	3,572	3,316
Montana	284	322	347	334	366	368	355	387	369	359
Nebraska	749	663	845	978	859	891	960	1,051	1,000	870
Nevada	199	268	215	256	281	268	283	319	300	322
New Hampshire	372	422	360	538	504	551	579	543	615	595
New Jersey	2,521	2,890	3,198	2,913	3,426	3,794	3,574	3,631	3,173	3,080
New Mexico	455	731	713	788	778	798	710	824	705	704
New York	9,401	9,122	10,638	10,861	10,735	11,678	12,571	13,942	14,570	12,997
North Carolina	2,920	2,881	3,526	3,753	3,599	3,597	3,833	4,141	3,817	3,919
North Dakota	225	191	301	374	341	381	320	406	312	382
Ohio	4,767	4,960	5,386	5,824	6,086	6,232	6,771	7,374	6,367	5,814
Oklahoma	1,244	1,335	1,350	1,513	1,642	1,761	1,657	1,710	1,712	1,629
Oregon	953	875	963	975	968	1,017	981	938	838	850
Pennsylvania	5,335	5,758	6,100	6,564	6,421	7,136	7,934	8,142	7,173	6,335
Rhode Island	440	402	382	486	579	886	902	673	662	568
South Carolina	1,031	1,239	1,387	1,579	1,763	1,742	1,673	1,778	1,703	1,752
South Dakota	629	542	365	486	473	561	579	554	535	417
Tennessee	2,179	2,848	2,702	3,025	2,940	3,191	3,440	3,654	3,250	2,950
Texas	4,758	5,631	6,880	6,905	7,273	7,851	7,533	7,344	7,282	7,093
Utah	345	450	507	810	523	680	719	685	666	590
Vermont	182	213	247	235	267	311	305	285	242	181
Virginia	2,035	2,149	2,597	2,551	2,665	3,151	3,030	3,027	2,975	2,807
Washington	1,769	1,544	1,770	1,547	1,552	1,527	1,704	1,626	1,486	1,550
West Virginia	1,001	915	1,052	1,033	1,120	1,140	1,185	1,133	1,116	1,068
Wisconsin	1,871	2,069	2,278	2,199	2,491	3,053	2,990	2,850	2,840	2,476
Wyoming	211	195	224	199	297	326	314	270	287	232
American Samoa	11	11	11	11	10	11	12	12	10	15
Guam	29	0	25	20	25	25	19	20	25	40
Puerto Rico	3,048	1,945	1,729	1,816	1,507	1,398	1,859	1,570	2,057	2,128
Virgin Islands	36	19	12	19	20	27	40	65	80	58

[1] National and regional totals exclude American Samoa, Guam, Puerto Rico, and the Virgin Islands.

29

Table 14
ANNUAL ADMISSIONS TO BASIC BACCALAUREATE NURSING PROGRAMS,
BY NLN REGION AND STATE: 1986-87 TO 1995-96[1]

NLN REGION AND STATE	NUMBER OF ADMISSIONS									
	1986-87	1987-88	1988-89	1989-90	1990-91	1991-92	1992-93	1993-94	1994-95	1995-96
United States	28,026	28,505	29,042	29,858	33,437	37,886	41,290	42,953	43,451	40,048
North Atlantic	6,545	6,449	6,525	6,412	6,549	7,612	9,845	9,746	9,673	9,240
Midwest	8,394	8,267	8,439	8,614	9,258	11,380	12,391	13,154	13,346	11,922
South	9,064	9,666	9,937	11,145	13,240	14,419	14,475	15,299	15,167	13,995
West	4,023	4,123	4,141	3,687	4,390	4,475	4,579	4,754	5,265	4,891
Alabama	976	834	853	915	821	1,096	1,086	1,091	1,143	1,101
Alaska	126	126	226	38	53	65	69	78	80	79
Arizona	279	270	287	191	270	285	337	347	452	471
Arkansas	289	310	321	317	447	426	471	591	478	429
California	1,746	1,720	1,595	1,371	1,769	1,802	1,696	1,768	2,298	1,872
Colorado	398	299	455	350	460	409	477	506	575	415
Connecticut	349	516	574	277	342	656	707	456	650	503
Delaware	117	117	122	88	72	188	278	256	283	174
D. of Columbia	255	359	225	199	279	263	491	293	311	275
Florida	714	652	770	779	915	925	1,015	940	1,010	1,020
Georgia	503	561	769	987	755	940	909	1,016	1,063	980
Hawaii	119	170	59	152	104	101	185	196	143	191
Idaho	44	78	87	69	85	74	90	90	90	130
Illinois	1,354	1,162	1,242	1,052	1,341	1,645	1,851	2,278	2,653	2,102
Indiana	1,082	1,116	1,092	995	1,188	1,271	1,362	1,338	1,455	1,474
Iowa	394	377	354	436	367	467	542	489	512	509
Kansas	353	403	428	523	507	643	899	694	664	577
Kentucky	554	607	662	566	815	738	635	785	811	690
Louisiana	790	911	1,009	1,247	2,184	1,925	1,708	2,086	1,978	1,216
Maine	205	226	311	283	338	196	426	237	425	294
Maryland	466	388	306	377	554	740	829	762	742	728
Massachusetts	823	715	785	1,134	998	1,180	1,190	1,227	1,171	1,174
Michigan	1,177	1,069	1,080	968	1,137	1,232	1,298	1,344	1,304	1,255
Minnesota	437	445	418	503	475	568	769	688	725	697
Mississippi	362	322	348	570	689	738	665	684	623	568
Missouri	569	601	557	528	702	1,019	967	1,262	1,537	1,364
Montana	176	220	187	221	239	233	224	258	235	225
Nebraska	608	538	610	648	499	572	617	745	644	541
Nevada	43	71	75	85	118	90	126	114	111	125
New Hampshire	110	81	99	136	151	168	175	162	152	171
New Jersey	528	681	408	386	397	459	422	562	478	472
New Mexico	55	77	74	145	227	192	40	128	160	193
New York	2,339	1,957	2,115	1,948	1,759	1,765	2,613	2,948	3,157	3,021
North Carolina	837	553	587	658	808	814	1,038	1,122	1,049	1,123
North Dakota	162	191	301	374	341	381	320	406	312	382
Ohio	1,265	1,219	1,282	1,507	1,447	1,916	2,077	2,272	1,966	1,771
Oklahoma	372	407	414	447	503	647	536	582	560	544
Oregon	370	288	286	327	369	434	378	376	318	337
Pennsylvania	1,611	1,618	1,738	1,724	1,931	2,080	2,903	3,259	2,730	2,838
Rhode Island	152	104	92	174	204	565	561	266	248	246
South Carolina	282	355	342	326	555	534	527	525	428	429
South Dakota	140	181	125	206	254	281	218	214	221	179
Tennessee	576	1,000	729	908	736	932	1,187	1,213	1,341	1,320
Texas	1,517	1,728	1,732	2,072	2,340	2,832	2,404	2,487	2,528	2,693
Utah	170	231	203	341	221	270	250	258	269	262
Vermont	56	75	56	63	78	92	79	80	68	72
Virginia	587	753	776	701	789	775	1,037	995	958	755
Washington	419	514	558	397	420	461	643	571	469	543
West Virginia	239	285	319	275	329	357	428	420	455	399
Wisconsin	853	965	950	874	1,000	1,385	1,471	1,424	1,353	1,071
Wyoming	78	59	49	0	55	59	64	64	65	48
American Samoa	0	0	0	0	0	0	0	0	0	0
Guam	0	0	25	20	25	25	19	20	25	40
Puerto Rico	2,335	1,301	996	900	672	686	786	804	910	973
Virgin Islands	18	9	7	5	10	18	25	42	52	33

[1] National and regional totals exclude American Samoa, Guam, Puerto Rico, and the Virgin Islands.

30

NLN REGION AND STATE	NUMBER OF ANNUAL ADMISSIONS									
	1986-87	1987-88	1988-89	1989-90	1990-91	1991-92	1992-93	1993-94	1994-95	1995-96
United States	54,330	57,375	63,973	68,634	69,869	74,079	75,382	77,343	76,016	72,930
North Atlantic	12,800	13,592	14,792	15,970	15,952	17,990	18,018	18,893	19,206	16,930
Midwest	13,974	13,927	15,652	16,888	17,503	18,117	18,369	19,356	18,952	18,746
South	18,894	20,695	23,753	25,816	26,940	28,170	28,864	29,071	28,391	27,545
West	8,662	9,161	9,776	9,960	9,474	9,802	10,131	10,023	9,467	9,709
Alabama	1,139	1,136	1,457	1,632	1,719	1,956	2,348	2,710	2,575	2,337
Alaska	40	40	40	43	50	37	36	32	28	32
Arizona	683	700	709	738	840	911	900	934	917	944
Arkansas	543	705	767	870	861	954	911	795	773	734
California	4,196	4,434	4,625	4,732	4,453	4,541	4,800	4,781	4,541	4,942
Colorado	544	574	637	576	551	611	587	535	523	516
Connecticut	442	457	356	472	512	672	478	413	467	470
Delaware	205	236	245	276	212	237	272	248	249	218
D. of Columbia	79	90	90	49	82	64	64	62	62	60
Florida	2,636	2,920	2,980	3,508	3,522	3,656	3,817	3,798	4,074	4,074
Georgia	1,215	1,420	1,432	1,738	1,811	2,063	2,343	2,350	2,235	1,910
Hawaii	64	175	213	209	177	200	224	199	194	190
Idaho	230	313	245	269	287	257	243	262	240	211
Illinois	2,723	2,418	3,024	3,032	3,247	3,342	3,139	3,244	3,459	3,534
Indiana	1,076	1,263	1,389	1,550	1,576	1,689	1,778	1,849	1,921	2,061
Iowa	1,006	1,124	1,111	1,114	1,237	1,293	1,466	1,582	1,499	1,492
Kansas	580	733	792	1,062	984	967	932	909	901	849
Kentucky	1,129	1,272	1,431	1,593	2,233	1,991	2,041	1,972	1,785	1,731
Louisiana	438	412	509	618	868	1,003	1,060	1,014	963	938
Maine	228	195	203	215	241	294	371	365	395	361
Maryland	899	927	1,079	1,061	1,098	1,220	1,235	1,324	1,265	1,324
Massachusetts	1,479	1,482	1,361	1,492	1,508	1,706	1,680	1,634	1,659	1,751
Michigan	2,451	2,298	2,348	2,584	2,458	2,763	2,586	2,647	2,692	2,636
Minnesota	994	1,125	1,370	1,436	1,284	1,406	1,273	1,309	1,190	1,185
Mississippi	1,141	1,118	1,236	1,418	1,400	1,406	1,519	1,527	1,494	1,587
Missouri	1,032	860	1,025	1,149	1,208	1,367	1,530	1,658	1,725	1,731
Montana	108	102	160	113	127	135	131	129	134	134
Nebraska	83	71	184	267	285	254	258	248	260	244
Nevada	156	197	140	171	163	178	157	205	189	197
New Hampshire	248	341	261	402	353	383	404	381	463	424
New Jersey	1,156	1,340	1,415	1,477	1,737	1,752	1,775	1,652	1,595	1,412
New Mexico	400	654	639	643	551	606	670	696	545	511
New York	6,592	6,743	8,013	8,453	8,494	9,496	9,643	10,761	11,116	9,767
North Carolina	1,969	2,150	2,414	2,741	2,501	2,499	2,513	2,666	2,541	2,570
North Dakota	63	0	0	0	0	0	0	0	0	0
Ohio	2,608	2,705	2,968	3,177	3,611	3,237	3,597	4,214	3,574	3,371
Oklahoma	872	928	936	1,066	1,139	1,114	1,121	1,128	1,152	1,085
Oregon	583	587	677	648	599	583	603	562	520	513
Pennsylvania	1,998	2,309	2,398	2,682	2,294	2,886	2,805	2,813	2,663	2,068
Rhode Island	247	261	259	280	330	281	300	359	363	290
South Carolina	740	884	1,045	1,253	1,208	1,208	1,146	1,253	1,275	1,323
South Dakota	385	305	217	280	219	280	361	340	314	238
Tennessee	1,301	1,432	1,462	1,630	1,767	1,771	1,675	1,649	1,507	1,371
Texas	3,111	3,764	4,948	4,641	4,725	4,779	4,898	4,625	4,519	4,204
Utah	175	219	304	469	302	410	469	427	397	328
Vermont	126	138	191	172	189	219	226	205	174	109
Virginia	1,150	1,077	1,406	1,374	1,377	1,854	1,566	1,625	1,634	1,688
Washington	1,350	1,030	1212	1,150	1,132	1,066	1,061	1,055	1,017	1.007
West Virginia	611	550	651	673	711	696	671	635	599	669
Wisconsin	973	1,025	1,224	1,237	1,394	1,519	1,449	1,356	1,417	1,405
Wyoming	133	136	175	199	242	267	250	206	222	184
American Samoa	11	11	11	11	10	11	12	12	10	15
Guam	29	0	0	0	0	0	0	0	0	0
Puerto Rico	713	644	733	916	835	712	1,073	766	1,147	1,155
Virgin Islands	18	10	5	14	10	9	15	23	28	25

[1] National and regional totals exclude American Samoa, Guam, Puerto Rico, and the Virgin Islands.

Table 16
ANNUAL ADMISSIONS TO DIPLOMA NURSING PROGRAMS,
BY NLN REGION AND STATE: 1986-87 TO 1995-96[1]

NLN REGION AND STATE	NUMBER OF ANNUAL ADMISSIONS									
	1986-87	1987-88	1988-89	1989-90	1990-91	1991-92	1992-93	1993-94	1994-95	1995-96
United States	8,337	8,389	10,010	10,088	10,220	10,691	10,165	9,601	7,717	6,227
North Atlantic	3,724	3,751	4,559	4,507	4,848	4,954	4,726	4,501	3,878	3,430
Midwest	2,783	2,453	2,771	2,908	2,841	3,030	2,819	2,330	1,927	1,392
South	1,674	2,019	2,393	2,436	2,288	2,473	2,425	2,609	1,753	1,405
West	156	166	287	237	243	234	195	161	159	0
Alabama	34	33	36	27	30	56	54	46	0	0
Alaska	0	0	0	0	0	0	0	0	0	0
Arizona	0	0	0	0	0	0	0	0	0	0
Arkansas	151	312	327	358	415	441	420	365	249	235
California	156	166	287	237	243	234	195	161	159	0
Colorado	0	0	0	0	0	0	0	0	0	0
Connecticut	221	227	270	321	287	185	185	180	174	122
Delaware	17	17	19	30	32	30	30	28	29	30
D. of Columbia	0	0	0	0	0	0	0	0	0	0
Florida	76	79	99	113	114	107	98	97	89	0
Georgia	87	94	88	0	0	0	0	0	0	0
Hawaii	0	0	0	0	0	0	0	0	0	0
Idaho	0	0	0	0	0	0	0	0	0	0
Illinois	345	260	358	369	301	297	327	252	204	216
Indiana	322	117	100	49	56	78	73	70	28	60
Iowa	261	167	207	302	334	386	410	287	268	86
Kansas	24	29	24	28	30	0	0	0	0	0
Kentucky	0	0	0	0	0	0	0	0	0	0
Louisiana	204	235	223	216	48	42	45	56	43	39
Maine	0	0	0	0	0	0	0	0	0	0
Maryland	118	134	157	128	167	206	204	183	63	86
Massachusetts	398	348	390	456	514	529	552	525	447	412
Michigan	244	154	154	196	295	313	255	245	124	52
Minnesota	0	0	0	0	0	0	0	0	0	0
Mississippi	0	0	0	0	0	0	0	0	0	0
Missouri	486	501	614	673	625	663	502	460	310	221
Montana	0	0	0	0	0	0	0	0	0	0
Nebraska	58	54	51	63	75	65	85	58	96	85
Nevada	0	0	0	0	0	0	0	0	0	0
New Hampshire	14	0	0	0	0	0	0	0	0	0
New Jersey	837	869	1,375	1,050	1,292	1,583	1,377	1,417	1,100	1,196
New Mexico	0	0	0	0	0	0	0	0	0	0
New York	470	422	510	460	482	417	315	233	297	209
North Carolina	114	178	255	354	290	284	282	353	227	226
North Dakota	0	0	0	0	0	0	0	0	0	0
Ohio	894	1,036	1,136	1,140	1,028	1,079	1,097	888	827	672
Oklahoma	0	0	0	0	0	0	0	0	0	0
Oregon	0	0	0	0	0	0	0	0	0	0
Pennsylvania	1,726	1,831	1,964	2,158	2,196	2,170	2,226	2,070	1,780	1,429
Rhode Island	41	37	31	32	45	40	41	48	51	32
South Carolina	9	0	0	0	0	0	0	0	0	0
South Dakota	104	56	23	0	0	0	0	0	0	0
Tennessee	302	416	511	487	437	488	578	792	402	259
Texas	130	139	200	192	208	240	231	232	235	196
Utah	0	0	0	0	0	0	0	0	0	0
Vermont	0	0	0	0	0	0	0	0	0	0
Virginia	298	319	415	476	499	522	427	407	383	364
Washington	0	0	0	0	0	0	0	0	0	0
West Virginia	151	80	82	85	80	87	86	78	62	0
Wisconsin	45	79	104	88	97	149	70	70	70	0
Wyoming	0	0	0	0	0	0	0	0	0	0
American Samoa	0	0	0	0	0	0	0	0	0	0
Guam	0	0	0	0	0	0	0	0	0	0
Puerto Rico	0	0	0	0	0	0	0	0	0	0
Virgin Islands	0	0	0	0	0	0	0	0	0	0

[1] National and regional totals exclude American Samoa, Guam, Puerto Rico, and the Virgin Islands.

Table 17
ENROLLMENTS IN BASIC RN PROGRAMS AND PERCENTAGE CHANGE
FROM PREVIOUS YEAR, BY TYPE OF PROGRAM: 1977 TO 1996[1]

YEAR	ALL BASIC RN PROGRAMS		BACCALAUREATE PROGRAMS		ASSOCIATE DEGREE PROGRAMS		DIPLOMA PROGRAMS	
	Number of Enrollments	Percent Change	Number of Enrollments	Percent Change	Number of Enrollments	Percent Change	Number of Enrollments	Percent Change
1977	245,390	-0.7	101,430	+1.5	91,102	+0.1	52,858	-5.8
1978	239,486	-2.4	99,900	-1.5	91,527	+0.5	48,059	-9.1
1979	234,659	-2.0	98,939	-1.0	92,069	+0.6	43,651	-9.2
1980	230,966	-1.6	95,858	-3.1	94,060	+2.2	41,048	-6.0
1981	234,995	+1.7	93,967	-2.0	100,019	+6.3	41,009	-0.1
1982	242,035	+3.0	94,363	+0.4	105,324	+5.3	42,348	+3.3
1983	250,553	+3.5	98,941	+4.9	109,605	+4.1	42,007	-0.8
1984	237,232	-5.3	95,008	-4.0	104,968	-4.2	37,256	-11.3
1985	217,955	-8.1	91,020	-4.2	96,756	-7.8	30,179	-19.0
1986	193,712	-11.1	81,602	-10.3	89,469	-7.5	22,641	-25.0
1987	182,947	-5.6	73,621	-9.8	90,399	+1.0	18,927	-16.4
1988	184,924	+1.1	70,078	-4.8	95,986	+6.2	18,860	-0.4
1989	201,458	+8.9	74,865	+6.8	106,175	+10.6	20,418	+8.3
1990	221,170	+9.8	81,788	+9.2	117,413	+10.6	21,969	+7.6
1991	237,598	+7.4	90,877	+11.1	123,816	+5.4	22,905	+4.3
1992	257,983	+8.6	102,128	+12.4	132,603	+7.1	23,252	+1.5
1993	270,228	+4.7	110,693	+8.4	137,300	+3.5	22,235	-4.4
1994	268,350	-0.7	112,659	+1.8	135,895	-1.0	19,796	-11.0
1995	261,219	-2.7	109,505	-2.8	135,235	-0.5	16,479	-16.8
1996	238,244	-8.8	103,213	-5.7	122,242	-9.6	12,789	-22.4

[1] Excludes American Samoa, Guam, Puerto Rico, and the Virgin Islands.

Table 18
ENROLLMENTS IN PUBLIC AND PRIVATE BASIC RN PROGRAMS, BY TYPE OF PROGRAM: 1987 TO 1996[1]

PUBLIC AND PRIVATE NURSING PROGRAMS	TOTAL ENROLLMENTS									
	1987	1988	1989	1990	1991	1992	1993	1994	1995	1996
All Programs	182,947	184,924	201,458	221,170	237,598	257,983	270,228	268,350	261,219	238,244
Public	130,230	134,575	148,343	162,707	176,892	186,230	193,951	191,193	176,828	162,806
Private	52,717	50,349	53,115	58,463	60,706	71,753	76,277	77,157	84,391	75,438
Baccalaureate	73,621	70,078	74,865	81,788	90,877	102,128	110,693	112,659	109,505	103,213
Public	47,276	45,414	49,792	54,245	59,257	62,045	65,643	65,331	62,514	59,061
Private	26,345	24,664	25,073	27,543	31,620	40,083	45,050	47,328	46,991	44,152
Assoc. Degree	90,399	95,986	106,175	117,413	123,816	132,603	137,300	135,895	135,235	122,242
Public	79,542	85,413	94,501	104,311	112,576	120,030	123,794	122,061	112,393	102,340
Private	10,857	10,573	11,674	13,102	11,240	12,573	13,506	13,834	22,842	19,902
Diploma	18,927	18,860	20,418	21,969	22,905	23,252	22,235	19,796	16,479	12,789
Public	3,412	3,748	4,050	4,151	5,059	4,155	4,514	3,801	1,921	1,405
Private	15,515	15,112	16,368	17,818	17,846	19,097	17,721	15,995	14,558	11,384

[1] Excludes American Samoa, Guam, Puerto Rico, and the Virgin Islands.

33

Table 19
TOTAL ENROLLMENTS IN ALL BASIC RN PROGRAMS, BY NLN REGION AND STATE: 1987 TO 1996[1]

NLN REGION AND STATE	NUMBER OF TOTAL ENROLLMENTS									
	1987	1988	1989	1990	1991	1992	1993	1994	1995	1996
United States	182,947	184,924	201,458	221,170	237,598	257,983	270,228	268,350	261,219	238,244
North Atlantic	50,521	49,533	53,315	56,673	60,276	68,512	72,271	74,088	75,344	63,043
Midwest	50,450	49,957	53,665	59,682	64,100	67,540	71,221	71,004	68,464	63,041
South	57,674	60,912	68,882	77,851	84,704	92,796	97,530	94,284	88,982	83,674
West	24,302	24,522	25,596	26,964	28,518	29,135	29,206	28,974	28,429	28,486
Alabama	3,799	4,003	4,462	4,886	5,704	6,962	8,008	8,380	7,637	6,713
Alaska	268	269	274	268	231	228	224	269	275	265
Arizona	1,827	1,819	1,765	1,799	1,881	2,095	2,350	2,309	2,363	2,363
Arkansas	1,929	2,170	2,627	3,268	3,628	3,734	3,534	3,347	2,880	2,650
California	12,108	11,668	12,003	12,455	13,511	13,599	13,526	13,525	13,074	13,242
Colorado	1,393	1,336	1,592	1,706	1,823	1,937	2,096	1,903	1,983	1,780
Connecticut	2,267	2,268	2,371	2,506	2,784	2,734	2,760	2,796	2,777	2,481
Delaware	829	800	879	937	809	1,155	1,327	1,332	1,228	1,117
D. of Columbia	754	799	704	710	759	877	983	1,051	1,141	908
Florida	5,475	5,877	6,371	7,181	7,800	8,166	8,510	8,918	8,809	8,453
Georgia	3,185	3,532	3,942	4,450	5,026	5,785	6,259	6,078	5,634	5,011
Hawaii	520	825	659	624	466	665	824	911	992	1,067
Idaho	550	625	710	885	722	684	692	704	670	700
Illinois	8,087	8,114	8,532	9,171	9,819	10,752	11,522	12,104	12,388	11,231
Indiana	5,830	6,007	6,219	7,916	8,027	6,871	7,093	7,370	7,594	6,216
Iowa	2,917	2,817	3,126	3,420	3,705	4,280	4,519	4,349	4,004	3,464
Kansas	1,791	1,951	2,272	2,721	2,725	3,015	3,125	3,072	2,870	2,840
Kentucky	3,550	3,801	4,250	4,515	5,527	5,914	5,663	5,594	5,177	4,584
Louisiana	4,957	5,462	7,163	7,620	7,604	10,336	12,240	10,130	9,212	8,830
Maine	1,001	984	1,153	1,350	1,508	1,827	1,969	1,934	1,628	1,774
Maryland	2,775	2,629	2,838	3,055	3,424	4,071	4,015	4,099	3,899	3,811
Massachusetts	6,239	5,593	6,232	6,513	7,062	7,883	8,313	8,334	8,147	7,549
Michigan	7,553	6,928	7,219	7,575	8,270	8,865	8,796	8,977	8,730	8,070
Minnesota	2,548	2,480	2,774	3,018	3,293	3,318	3,521	3,357	3,228	3,130
Mississippi	2,584	2,720	2,980	3,488	3,658	3,974	3,995	3,761	3,623	3,543
Missouri	3,875	3,702	3,943	4,421	5,032	5,956	6,337	6,017	6,018	5,618
Montana	739	868	896	916	888	994	974	915	885	858
Nebraska	1,169	1,196	1,603	2,011	2,369	2,535	2,552	2,458	2,273	2,127
Nevada	488	439	452	568	638	490	556	513	534	634
New Hampshire	803	805	905	1,116	1,243	1,408	1,422	1,418	1,369	1,246
New Jersey	5,410	5,642	5,959	6,418	7,140	7,788	7,886	7,698	7,079	6,212
New Mexico	920	987	1,072	1,220	1,337	1,386	1,347	1,428	1,310	1,272
New York	19,266	18,105	19,414	20,056	21,110	24,515	26,656	28,916	33,368	26,101
North Carolina	4,679	5,086	5,852	6,677	6,721	7,000	7,304	7,251	7,135	6,894
North Dakota	650	551	738	862	722	913	808	777	732	707
Ohio	10,651	10,748	11,464	11,866	12,523	13,450	14,218	14,487	13,372	12,494
Oklahoma	2,324	2,243	2,562	2,840	3,241	3,363	3,345	3,251	3,130	3,002
Oregon	1,620	1,595	1,747	1,851	2,012	1,967	1,480	1,680	1,642	1,683
Pennsylvania	12,325	13,106	14,159	15,294	15,776	18,069	18,596	18,009	16,179	13,820
Rhode Island	1,213	1,017	1,086	1,258	1,482	1,584	1,678	1,951	1,893	1,414
South Carolina	2,424	2,664	2,931	3,658	3,383	4,026	3,891	3,764	3,595	3,592
South Dakota	1,104	1,057	1,125	1,071	1,653	1,255	1,255	1,112	1,092	1,060
Tennessee	4,797	4,726	4,981	6,56	6,836	6,167	6,830	6,724	6,240	5,758
Texas	9,313	10,082	11,394	12,366	14,004	14,360	15,087	14,089	13,496	12,742
Utah	794	779	1,003	1,066	1,093	1,250	1,299	1,192	1,109	1,248
Vermont	414	414	453	515	603	672	681	649	535	421
Virginia	4,045	4,139	4,577	5,186	5,810	6,414	6,178	6,260	6,236	5,821
Washington	2,633	2,828	2,945	3,044	3,211	3,246	3,288	3,146	3,111	2,947
West Virginia	1,838	1,778	1,952	2,095	2,338	2,524	2,671	2,638	2,279	2,270
Wisconsin	4,275	4,406	4,650	5,630	5,962	6,330	7,475	6,924	6,163	6,084
Wyoming	442	484	478	562	705	594	550	479	481	427
American Samoa	16	16	16	16	13	16	11	11	15	21
Guam	60	0	19	20	69	69	68	113	102	80
Puerto Rico	3,561	2,918	2,980	3,408	3,120	3,575	4,157	3,754	4,354	4,347
Virgin Islands	73	50	47	55	55	75	77	111	111	133

[1] National and regional totals exclude American Samoa, Guam, Puerto Rico, and the Virgin Islands.

Table 20
TOTAL ENROLLMENTS IN BASIC BACCALAUREATE NURSING PROGRAMS,
BY NLN REGION AND STATE: 1987 TO 1996[1]

NLN REGION AND STATE	N U M B E R O F T O T A L E N R O L L M E N T S[2]									
	1987	1988	1989	1990	1991	1992	1993	1994	1995	1996
United States	73,621	70,078	74,865	81,788	90,877	102,128	110,693	112,659	109,505	103,213
North Atlantic	19,710	17,695	17,742	18,563	20,450	24,777	27,797	28,628	27,686	25,064
Midwest	21,823	21,183	21,916	24,164	27,762	29,691	32,253	33,649	32,714	30,910
South	22,564	22,134	25,846	28,978	31,823	36,418	39,622	38,817	37,018	35,279
West	9,524	9,066	9,361	10,083	10,842	11,242	11,021	11,565	12,087	11,960
Alabama	1,991	1,904	2,040	2,160	2,723	3,546	4,040	4,070	3,734	3,193
Alaska	203	203	199	182	151	156	156	212	220	207
Arizona	591	595	546	523	548	644	801	843	877	866
Arkansas	580	549	672	740	856	969	1,091	1,229	884	886
California	4,309	3,947	3,990	4,173	4,654	4,747	4,676	4,855	4,962	4,916
Colorado	711	585	756	871	963	1,111	1,108	981	1,112	981
Connecticut	1,076	1,012	988	1,136	1,114	1,260	1,420	1,463	1,534	1,421
Delaware	467	411	419	460	343	633	759	819	719	652
D. of Columbia	675	647	552	564	669	801	886	955	1,045	833
Florida	1,430	1,418	1,494	1,567	1,809	2,020	1,873	2,328	2,436	2,304
Georgia	901	988	1,215	1,372	1,589	1,810	2,136	2,249	2,261	2,208
Hawaii	401	354	284	162	220	288	429	548	696	762
Idaho	107	183	223	369	189	187	209	215	217	287
Illinois	3,249	3,059	3,028	3,131	3,667	4,201	4,787	5,977	6,020	5,460
Indiana	3,351	3,418	3,321	4,155	4,711	3,344	3,441	3,614	3,685	3,023
Iowa	821	779	788	859	1,006	1,182	1,308	1,338	1,320	1,266
Kansas	780	836	940	1,137	1,230	1,520	1,549	1,613	1,472	1,484
Kentucky	1,477	1,571	1,846	1,721	2,191	2,304	1,934	2,013	1,985	1,741
Louisiana	3,361	3,623	5,127	5,595	5,214	7,465	8,530	7,280	6,596	6,501
Maine	700	666	797	912	1,018	1,157	1,313	1,305	1,024	1,174
Maryland	968	758	819	770	974	1,244	1,385	1,543	1,525	1,579
Massachusetts	2,970	2,578	2,821	2,770	3,030	3,599	3,887	4,000	4,003	3,825
Michigan	3,157	3,096	2,867	2,991	3,341	3,717	3,582	3,699	3,816	3,838
Minnesota	1,046	844	895	903	1,072	1,140	1,307	1,159	1,178	1,153
Mississippi	998	958	995	1,311	1,428	1,494	1,399	1,170	1,063	1,020
Missouri	1,217	1,057	1,035	1,329	1,778	2,610	2,850	2,527	2,897	2,923
Montana	565	606	621	672	648	749	741	622	670	640
Nebraska	824	1,026	1,295	1,514	1,808	1,914	1,929	1,872	1,698	1,521
Nevada	193	231	281	338	376	255	267	271	266	290
New Hampshire	363	329	352	389	482	523	567	582	530	500
New Jersey	1,480	1,056	1,251	1,313	1,424	1,590	1,662	1,672	1,588	1,472
New Mexico	190	181	174	208	318	377	329	352	431	432
New York	5,793	4,981	4,603	4,389	5,000	6,469	7,701	8,158	8,154	7,299
North Carolina	1,563	1,348	1,409	1,776	1,745	2,081	2,265	2,239	2,287	2,010
North Dakota	537	551	738	862	722	913	808	777	732	707
Ohio	3,781	3,571	3,789	3,950	4,210	5,137	5,696	6,313	5,723	5,342
Oklahoma	933	780	947	1,076	1,271	1,357	1,266	1,233	1,242	1,133
Oregon	665	616	666	745	905	922	412	773	726	717
Pennsylvania	5,288	5,364	5,330	5,812	6,327	7,528	8,286	8,405	7,878	6,752
Rhode Island	682	470	461	616	809	966	1,060	1,019	946	893
South Carolina	994	997	1,049	1,139	1,337	1,777	1,753	1,774	1,618	1,556
South Dakota	594	555	632	606	1,165	744	592	554	609	563
Tennessee	1,667	1,629	1,662	2,547	2,418	1,868	2,544	2,761	2,806	2,592
Texas	3,747	3,676	4,238	4,492	5,350	5,224	5,890	5,371	5,256	5,173
Utah	395	378	415	523	442	515	544	576	577	576
Vermont	216	181	168	202	234	251	256	250	265	243
Virginia	1,339	1,327	1,611	1,850	1,911	2,165	2,255	2,255	2,235	2,254
Washington	977	962	971	1,079	1,179	1,166	1,227	1,194	1,218	1,191
West Virginia	615	608	722	862	1,007	1,094	1,261	1,302	1,090	1,129
Wisconsin	2,466	2,391	2,588	2,727	3,052	3,269	4,404	4,206	3,564	3,630
Wyoming	217	225	235	238	249	125	122	123	115	95
American Samoa	0	0	0	0	0	0	0	0	0	0
Guam	0	0	19	20	69	69	68	113	102	80
Puerto Rico	2,615	2,118	1,873	1,952	1,672	1,937	2,213	2,236	2,403	2,509
Virgin Islands	46	27	26	38	41	54	41	80	71	72

[1]National and regional totals exclude American Samoa, Guam, Puerto Rico, and the Virgin Islands.
[2]Includes basic students only.

Table 21
TOTAL ENROLLMENTS IN ASSOCIATE DEGREE NURSING PROGRAMS, BY NLN REGION AND STATE: 1987 TO 1996[1]

NLN REGION AND STATE	NUMBER OF TOTAL ENROLLMENTS									
	1987	1988	1989	1990	1991	1992	1993	1994	1995	1996
United States	90,399	95,986	106,175	117,413	123,816	132,603	137,300	135,895	135,235	122,242
North Atlantic	22,296	23,044	25,932	27,695	28,983	32,747	34,038	35,660	39,190	31,059
Midwest	22,497	23,215	26,084	29,737	30,330	31,590	32,876	32,385	31,644	29,135
South	31,166	34,576	38,281	43,550	47,296	50,835	52,583	50,773	48,304	45,522
West	14,440	15,151	15,878	16,431	17,207	17,431	17,803	17,077	16,097	16,526
Alabama	1,742	2,039	2,363	2,648	2,881	3,319	3,885	4,281	3,903	3,520
Alaska	65	66	75	86	80	72	68	57	55	58
Arizona	1,236	1,224	1,219	1,276	1,333	1,451	1,549	1,466	1,486	1,497
Arkansas	927	997	1,225	1,486	1,591	1,542	1,499	1,381	1,353	1,237
California	7,461	7,416	7,656	7,832	8,388	8,390	8,468	8,338	7,867	8,326
Colorado	682	751	836	835	860	826	988	922	871	799
Connecticut	680	703	761	638	1,038	1,113	970	976	966	890
Delaware	320	343	417	427	408	449	493	440	437	399
D. of Columbia	79	152	152	146	90	76	97	96	96	75
Florida	3,905	4,299	4,672	5,383	5,799	5,966	6,446	6,399	6,247	6,149
Georgia	2,045	2,323	2,584	3,010	3,419	3,975	4,123	3,829	3,373	2,803
Hawaii	119	471	375	462	246	377	395	363	296	305
Idaho	443	442	487	516	533	497	483	489	453	413
Illinois	4,020	4,349	4,835	5,359	5,524	5,806	5,955	5,479	5,773	5,255
Indiana	1,969	2,339	2,695	3,604	3,125	3,297	3,363	3,493	3,709	3,039
Iowa	1,685	1,603	1,808	1,910	1,929	2,161	2,323	2,294	2,027	1,864
Kansas	947	1,063	1,269	1,512	1,446	1,465	1,576	1,459	1,398	1,356
Kentucky	2,073	2,230	2,404	2,794	3,336	3,610	3,729	3,581	3,192	2,843
Louisiana	993	1,260	1,510	1,676	2,168	2,797	3,633	2,769	2,536	2,264
Maine	284	318	356	438	490	670	656	629	604	600
Maryland	1,574	1,608	1,714	1,953	2,104	2,473	2,272	2,246	2,135	2,072
Massachusetts	2,328	2,274	2,560	2,718	2,876	3,068	3,202	3,148	3,058	2,840
Michigan	4,020	3,495	4,009	4,217	4,504	4,679	4,729	4,866	4,755	4,139
Minnesota	1,502	1,636	1,879	2,115	2,221	2,178	2,214	2,198	2,050	1,977
Mississippi	1,586	1,762	1,985	2,177	2,230	2,480	2,596	2,591	2,560	2,523
Missouri	1,567	1,561	1,664	1,857	2,032	2,260	2,479	2,689	2,542	2,365
Montana	174	262	275	244	240	245	233	293	215	218
Nebraska	156	97	232	414	478	520	498	483	458	479
Nevada	295	208	171	230	262	235	289	242	268	344
New Hampshire	401	467	553	727	761	885	855	836	839	746
New Jersey	2,048	2,280	2,311	2,455	2,707	2,932	2,946	2,909	2,709	2,429
New Mexico	730	806	898	1,012	1,019	1,009	1,018	1,076	879	840
New York	12,339	12,151	13,710	14,555	15,132	17,154	18,417	20,263	24,784	18,479
North Carolina	2,789	3,362	3,877	4,238	4,313	4,262	4,311	4,337	4,382	4,427
North Dakota	85	0	0	0	0	0	0	0	0	0
Ohio	4,478	4,826	5,332	5,580	5,900	5,933	6,311	6,283	5,967	5,767
Oklahoma	1,391	1,463	1,615	1,764	1,970	2,006	2,079	2,018	1,888	1,869
Oregon	955	979	1,081	1,106	1,107	1,045	1,068	907	916	966
Pennsylvania	3,202	3,659	4,280	4,722	4,536	5,463	5,468	5,146	4,584	4,007
Rhode Island	417	464	547	556	576	516	509	818	843	416
South Carolina	1,421	1,667	1,882	2,519	2,046	2,249	2,138	1,990	1,977	2,036
South Dakota	414	383	445	444	488	511	663	558	483	497
Tennessee	2,302	2,381	2,476	3,046	3,292	3,118	3,102	2,920	2,714	2,655
Texas	5,340	6,142	6,830	7,482	8,225	8,698	8,760	8,297	7,857	7,231
Utah	399	401	588	543	651	735	755	616	532	672
Vermont	198	233	285	313	369	421	425	399	270	178
Virginia	2,015	2,038	2,075	2,299	2,743	3,061	2,755	2,935	3,058	2,756
Washington	1,656	1,866	1974	1,965	2,032	2,080	2,061	1,952	1,893	1,756
West Virginia	1,063	1,005	1,069	1,075	1,179	1,279	1,255	1,199	1,129	1,137
Wisconsin	1,654	1,863	1,916	2,725	2,683	2,780	2,765	2,583	2,482	2,397
Wyoming	225	259	243	324	456	469	428	356	366	332
American Samoa	16	16	16	16	13	16	11	11	15	21
Guam	60	0	0	0	0	0	0	0	0	0
Puerto Rico	946	800	1,107	1,456	1,448	1,638	1,944	1,518	1,951	1,838
Virgin Islands	27	23	21	17	14	21	36	31	40	61

[1] National and regional totals exclude American Samoa, Guam, Puerto Rico, and the Virgin Islands.

NLN REGION AND STATE	NUMBER OF TOTAL ENROLLMENTS									
	1987	1988	1989	1990	1991	1992	1993	1994	1995	1996
United States	18,927	18,860	20,418	21,969	22,905	23,252	22,235	19,796	16,479	12,789
North Atlantic	8,515	8,794	9,641	10,415	10,843	10,988	10,436	9,800	8,468	6,920
Midwest	6,130	5,559	5,665	5,781	6,008	6,259	6,092	4,970	4,106	2,996
South	3,944	4,202	4,755	5,323	5,585	5,543	5,325	4,694	3,660	2,873
West	338	305	357	450	469	462	382	332	245	0
Alabama	66	60	59	78	100	97	83	29	0	0
Alaska	0	0	0	0	0	0	0	0	0	0
Arizona	0	0	0	0	0	0	0	0	0	0
Arkansas	422	624	730	1,042	1,181	1,223	944	737	643	527
California	338	305	357	450	469	462	382	332	245	0
Colorado	0	0	0	0	0	0	0	0	0	0
Connecticut	511	553	622	732	632	361	370	357	277	170
Delaware	42	46	43	50	58	73	75	73	72	66
D. of Columbia	0	0	0	0	0	0	0	0	0	0
Florida	140	160	205	231	192	180	191	191	126	0
Georgia	239	221	143	68	18	0	0	0	0	0
Hawaii	0	0	0	0	0	0	0	0	0	0
Idaho	0	0	0	0	0	0	0	0	0	0
Illinois	818	706	669	681	628	745	780	648	595	516
Indiana	510	250	203	157	191	230	289	263	200	154
Iowa	411	435	530	651	770	937	888	717	65	334
Kansas	64	52	63	72	49	30	0	0	0	0
Kentucky	0	0	0	0	0	0	0	0	0	0
Louisiana	603	579	526	349	222	74	77	81	80	65
Maine	17	0	0	0	0	0	0	0	0	0
Maryland	233	263	305	332	346	354	358	310	239	160
Massachusetts	941	741	851	1,025	1,156	1,216	1,224	1,186	1,086	884
Michigan	376	337	343	367	425	469	485	412	159	93
Minnesota	0	0	0	0	0	0	0	0	0	0
Mississippi	0	0	0	0	0	0	0	0	0	0
Missouri	1,091	1,084	1,244	1,235	1,222	1,086	1,008	801	579	330
Montana	0	0	0	0	0	0	0	0	0	0
Nebraska	189	73	76	83	83	101	125	103	117	127
Nevada	0	0	0	0	0	0	0	0	0	0
New Hampshire	39	9	0	0	0	0	0	0	0	0
New Jersey	1,882	2,306	2,397	2,650	3,009	3,266	3,278	3,117	2,782	2,311
New Mexico	0	0	0	0	0	0	0	0	0	0
New York	1,134	973	1,101	1,112	978	892	538	495	430	323
North Carolina	327	376	566	663	663	657	728	675	466	457
North Dakota	28	0	0	0	0	0	0	0	0	0
Ohio	2,392	2,351	2,343	2,336	2,413	2,380	2,211	1,891	1,682	1,385
Oklahoma	0	0	0	0	0	0	0	0	0	0
Oregon	0	0	0	0	0	0	0	0	0	0
Pennsylvania	3,835	4,083	4,549	4,760	4,913	5,078	4,842	4,458	3,717	3,061
Rhode Island	114	83	78	86	97	102	109	114	104	105
South Carolina	9	0	0	0	0	0	0	0	0	0
South Dakota	96	119	48	21	0	0	0	0	0	0
Tennessee	828	716	843	973	1,126	1,181	1,184	1,043	720	511
Texas	226	264	326	392	429	438	437	421	383	338
Utah	0	0	0	0	0	0	0	0	0	0
Vermont	0	0	0	0	0	0	0	0	0	0
Virginia	691	774	891	1,037	1,156	1,188	1,168	1,070	943	811
Washington	0	0	0	0	0	0	0	0	0	0
West Virginia	160	165	161	158	152	151	155	137	60	4
Wisconsin	155	152	146	178	227	281	306	135	117	57
Wyoming	0	0	0	0	0	0	0	0	0	0
American Samoa	0	0	0	0	0	0	0	0	0	0
Guam	0	0	0	0	0	0	0	0	0	0
Puerto Rico	0	0	0	0	0	0	0	0	0	0
Virgin Islands	0	0	0	0	0	0	0	0	0	0

[1] National and regional totals exclude American Samoa, Guam, Puerto Rico, and the Virgin Islands.

Table 23
BASIC AND RN STUDENT ENROLLMENTS IN BACCALAUREATE NURSING PROGRAMS:
1987 TO 1996[1]

YEAR	ENROLLMENTS IN BACCALAUREATE NURSING PROGRAMS			
	Total Enrollments	Basic Programs		BRN* Programs
		Basic Students	RN Students	RN Students
1987	119,996	73,621	26,503	19,872
1988	113,105	70,078	25,597	17,430
1989	116,539	74,865	24,524	17,150
1990	122,504	81,788	23,777	16,939
1991	130,195	90,877	22,634	16,684
1992	142,494	102,128	22,399	17,967
1993	151,566	110,693	23,075	17,798
1994	155,655	112,659	25,536	17,460
1995	156,605	109,505	26,057	21,043
1996	151,243	103,213	27,408	20,622

[1] Excludes American Samoa, Guam, Puerto Rico, and the Virgin Islands.
* BRN programs are baccalaureate programs that admit only RNs.

Table 24
FULL-TIME AND PART-TIME ENROLLMENTS OF BASIC AND RN STUDENTS
IN BACCALAUREATE NURSING PROGRAMS: 1992 TO 1996[1]

YEAR AND TYPE OF STUDENT	ENROLLMENTS IN BACCALAUREATE NURSING PROGRAMS		
	Total	Full-Time	Part-Time
1992 (Total)	142,494	95,745	46,749
Basic Students	102,128	88,002	14,126
RNs in Basic Programs	22,399	4,353	18,046
RNs in BRN* Programs	17,967	3,390	14,577
1993 (Total)	151,566	104,793	46,773
Basic Students	110,693	96,316	14,377
RNs in Basic Programs	23,075	4,617	18,458
RNs in BRN* Programs	17,798	3,860	13,938
1994 (Total)	155,655	105,021	50,634
Basic Students	112,659	96,653	16,006
RNs in Basic Programs	25,536	4,549	20,987
RNs in BRN* Programs	17,460	3,819	13,641
1995 (Total)	156,605	104,413	52,192
Basic Students	109,505	94,797	14,708
RNs in Basic Programs	26,057	4,649	21,408
RNs in BRN* Programs	21,043	4,967	16,076
1996 (Total)	151,243	99,561	51,682
Basic Students	103,213	88,832	14,381
RNs in Basic Programs	27,408	5,313	22,095
RNs in BRN* Programs	20,622	5,416	15,206

[1] Excludes American Samoa, Guam, Puerto Rico, and the Virgin Islands.
* BRN programs are baccalaureate programs that admit only RNs.

Table 25
TOTAL ENROLLMENTS IN BACCALAUREATE NURSING PROGRAMS, BY NLN REGION AND STATE:
1992 TO 1996[1]

NLN REGION AND STATE	ENROLLMENTS IN BACCALAUREATE NURSING PROGRAMS[2]									
	1992		1993		1994		1995		1996	
	Total	RNs Only	Total	RNs Only	Total	RNs Only	Total	RNs Only	Total	RNs Only
United States	142,494	40,366	151,566	40,873	155,655	42,996	156,605	47,100	151,243	48,030
North Atlantic	39,973	15,196	43,267	15,470	46,490	17,862	46,399	18,713	44,408	19,344
Midwest	40,577	10,886	43,225	10,972	45,071	11,422	44,317	11,603	42,736	11,826
South	44,153	7,735	47,651	8,029	47,656	8,839	46,989	9,971	45,136	9,857
West	17,791	6,549	17,423	6,402	16,438	4,873	18,900	6,813	18,963	7,003
Alabama	3,969	423	4,424	384	4,501	431	4,269	535	3,693	500
Alaska	167	11	165	9	222	10	227	7	255	48
Arizona	1,767	1,123	2,062	1,261	2,350	1,507	2,718	1,841	3,083	2,217
Arkansas	1,072	103	1,188	97	1,366	137	973	89	982	96
California	8,197	3,450	7,988	3,312	5,990	1,135	7,815	2,853	7,583	2,667
Colorado	1,602	491	1,642	534	1,594	613	1,714	602	1,465	484
Connecticut	1,963	703	2,182	762	2,415	952	2,466	932	2,206	785
Delaware	996	363	1,289	530	1,545	726	1,513	794	1,243	591
D. of Columbia	916	115	968	82	1,032	77	1,106	61	903	70
Florida	3,247	1,227	3,229	1,356	3,868	1,540	3,960	1,524	4,068	1,764
Georgia	2,313	503	2,702	566	2,879	630	2,962	701	2,886	678
Hawaii	422	134	562	133	673	1257	786	90	827	65
Idaho	310	123	339	130	339	124	258	41	512	225
Illinois	5,703	1,502	6,176	1,389	7,466	1,489	7,569	1,549	7,243	1,783
Indiana	4,360	1,016	4,427	986	4,694	1,080	5,047	1,362	4,396	1,373
Iowa	2,043	861	2,311	1,003	1,876	538	1,845	525	1,828	562
Kansas	2,151	631	2,148	599	2,234	621	1,758	286	1,893	409
Kentucky	2,825	521	2,494	560	2,456	443	2,523	538	2,189	448
Louisiana	7,803	338	8,867	337	7,694	414	7,060	464	6,918	417
Maine	1,575	418	1,825	512	1,872	567	1,681	657	1,896	722
Maryland	1,939	695	1,995	610	2,170	627	2,354	829	2,405	826
Massachusetts	5,261	1,662	5,177	1,290	5,820	1,820	5,836	1,833	5,403	1,578
Michigan	5,354	1,637	5,187	1,605	5,101	1,402	5,347	1,531	5,110	1,272
Minnesota	1,706	566	1,875	568	1,775	616	1,791	613	1,834	681
Mississippi	1,573	79	1,515	116	1,368	198	1,260	197	1,226	206
Missouri	3,941	1,331	4,148	1,298	4,470	1,943	4,874	1,977	5,339	2,416
Montana	783	34	770	29	727	105	766	96	678	38
Nebraska	2,376	462	2,430	501	2,256	384	2,197	499	1,830	309
Nevada	302	47	311	44	308	37	305	39	323	33
New Hampshire	744	221	826	259	1,212	630	1,110	580	1,140	640
New Jersey	2,932	1,342	3,020	1,358	3,301	1,629	3,444	1,856	3,538	2,066
New Mexico	639	262	593	264	626	274	797	366	774	342
New York	12,938	6,469	14,378	6,677	14,916	6,758	15,618	7,464	15,085	7,786
North Carolina	2,793	712	3,005	740	3,059	820	3,256	969	2,903	893
North Dakota	974	61	859	51	877	100	839	107	810	103
Ohio	7,011	1,874	7,486	1,790	8,376	2,063	7,739	2,016	7,148	1,806
Oklahoma	1,501	144	1,403	137	1,393	160	1,405	163	1,277	144
Oregon	1,123	201	431	19	958	185	893	167	889	172
Pennsylvania	11,089	3,561	11,968	3,682	12,808	4,403	12,154	4,276	11,614	4,862
Rhode Island	1,122	156	1,169	109	1,152	133	997	51	984	91
South Carolina	2,026	249	2,053	300	2,064	290	1,976	358	1,900	344
South Dakota	872	128	825	233	673	119	710	101	637	74
Tennessee	2,472	604	3,171	627	3,481	720	3,439	633	3,087	495
Texas	6,156	932	6,939	1,049	6,365	994	6,162	906	6,103	930
Utah	732	217	803	259	833	257	809	232	828	252
Vermont	437	186	465	209	417	167	474	209	396	153
Virginia	2,896	731	2,993	738	3,212	957	3,862	1,627	3,970	1,716
Washington	1,615	449	1,627	400	1,683	489	1,666	448	1,615	424
West Virginia	1,568	474	1,673	412	1,780	478	1,528	438	1,529	400
Wisconsin	4,086	817	5,353	949	5,273	1,067	4,601	1,037	4,668	1,038
Wyoming	132	7	130	8	135	12	146	31	131	36
American Samoa	0	0	0	0	0	0	0	0	0	0
Guam	69	0	79	11	123	10	107	5	89	9
Puerto Rico	2,253	316	2,471	258	2,517	281	2,685	282	2,790	281
Virgin Islands	60	6	45	4	91	11	73	2	74	2

[1] National and regional totals exclude American Samoa, Guam, Puerto Rico, and the Virgin Islands.
[2] Totals include RNs in basic programs, RNs in BRN programs, and basic BSN students.

Table 26

GRADUATIONS FROM BASIC RN PROGRAMS AND PERCENTAGE CHANGE
FROM PREVIOUS YEAR, BY TYPE OF PROGRAM: 1976-77 TO 1995-96[1]

ACADEMIC YEAR	ALL BASIC RN PROGRAMS		BACCALAUREATE PROGRAMS		ASSOCIATE DEGREE PROGRAMS		DIPLOMA PROGRAMS	
	Number of Graduations	Percent Change	Number of Graduations	Percent Change	Number of Graduations	Percent Change	Number of Graduations	Percent Change
1976-77	77,755	+0.9	23,452	+3.9	36,289	+4.8	18,014	-9.3
1977-78	77,874	+0.1	24,187	+3.1	36,556	+0.7	17,131	-4.9
1978-79	77,132	-1.0	25,048	+3.6	36,264	-0.8	15,820	-7.7
1979-80	75,523	-2.1	24,994	-0.2	36,034	-0.6	14,495	-8.4
1980-81	73,985	-2.0	24,370	-2.5	36,712	+1.9	12,903	-11.0
1981-82	74,052	+0.1	24,081	-1.2	38,289	+4.3	11,682	-9.5
1982-83	77,408	+4.5	23,855	-0.9	41,849	+9.3	11,704	+0.2
1983-84	80,312	+3.8	23,718	-0.6	44,394	+6.1	12,200	+4.2
1984-85	82,075	+2.2	24,975	+5.3	45,208	+1.8	11,892	-2.5
1985-86	77,027	-6.2	25,170	+0.8	41,333	-8.6	10,524	-11.5
1986-87	70,561	-8.4	23,761	-5.6	38,528	-6.8	8,272	-21.4
1987-88	64,839	-8.0	21,504	-9.5	37,397	-2.9	5,938	-28.2
1988-89	61,660	-4.9	18,997	-11.6	37,837	+1.2	4,826	-18.7
1989-90	66,088	+7.2	18,571	-2.2	42,318	+11.8	5,199	+7.7
1990-91	72,230	+9.3	19,264	+3.7	46,794	+10.6	6,172	+18.7
1991-92	80,839	+11.9	21,415	+11.2	52,896	+13.0	6,528	+5.8
1992-93	88,149	+9.0	24,442	+14.1	56,770	+7.3	6,937	+6.3
1993-94	94,870	+7.6	28,912	+18.3	58,839	+3.6	7,119	+2.6
1994-95	97,052	+2.3	31,254	+8.1	58,749	-0.1	7,049	-1.0
1995-96	94,757	-2.4	32,413	+3.7	56,641	-3.6	5,703	-19.1

[1] Excludes American Samoa, Guam, Puerto Rico, and the Virgin Islands.

Table 27

GRADUATIONS FROM PUBLIC AND PRIVATE BASIC RN PROGRAMS, BY TYPE OF PROGRAM: 1986-87 TO 1995-96[1]

PUBLIC AND PRIVATE NURSING PROGRAMS	NUMBER OF GRADUATIONS									
	1986-87	1987-88	1988-89	1989-90	1990-91	1991-92	1992-93	1993-94	1994-95	1995-96
All Programs	70,561	64,839	61,660	66,088	72,230	80,839	88,149	94,870	97,052	94,757
Public	50,865	48,608	47,644	51,926	57,892	64,405	70,152	73,610	71,841	69,199
Private	19,696	16,231	14,016	14,162	14,338	16,434	17,997	21,260	25,211	25,558
Baccalaureate	23,761	21,504	18,997	18,571	19,264	21,415	24,442	28,912	31,254	32,413
Public	14,746	13,568	12,203	12,434	13,073	14,498	16,588	18,902	19,427	19,417
Private	9,015	7,936	6,794	6,137	6,191	6,917	7,854	10,010	11,827	12,996
Assoc. Degree	38,528	37,397	37,837	42,318	46,794	52,896	56,770	58,839	58,749	56,641
Public	34,696	33,795	34,460	38,439	43,337	48,535	52,017	53,294	51,448	49,140
Private	3,832	3,602	3,377	3,879	3,457	4,361	4,753	5,545	7,301	7,501
Diploma	8,272	5,938	4,826	5,199	6,172	6,528	6,937	7,119	7,049	5,703
Public	1,423	1,245	981	1,053	1,482	1,372	1,547	1,414	966	642
Private	6,849	4,693	3,845	4,146	4,690	5,156	5,390	5,705	6,083	5,061

[1] Excludes American Samoa, Guam, Puerto Rico, and the Virgin Islands.

Table 28
GRADUATIONS FROM ALL BASIC RN PROGRAMS, BY NLN REGION AND STATE: 1986-87 TO 1995-96[1]

NLN REGION AND STATE	NUMBER OF GRADUATIONS									
	1986-87	1987-88	1988-89	1989-90	1990-91	1991-92	1992-93	1993-94	1994-95	1995-96
United States	70,561	64,839	61,660	66,088	72,230	80,839	88,149	94,870	97,052	94,757
North Atlantic	18,274	16,617	15,054	15,347	16,278	18,762	20,116	21,414	22,484	22,371
Midwest	20,664	18,072	17,264	18,354	19,961	21,900	24,137	25,713	26,865	26,149
South	21,397	20,123	19,768	21,982	25,214	28,622	32,047	35,133	35,552	33,983
West	10,226	10,027	9,574	10,405	10,777	11,555	11,849	12,610	12,151	12,254
Alabama	1,587	1,430	1,354	1,425	1,565	1,867	1,970	2,642	2,843	2,758
Alaska	51	46	64	62	51	77	78	79	74	95
Arizona	795	767	784	807	796	792	918	1,064	1,066	1,057
Arkansas	726	685	687	878	1,039	1,224	1,216	1,254	1,252	1,202
California	5,125	4,969	4,716	4,956	5,045	5,245	5,295	5,591	5,431	5,371
Colorado	521	552	524	584	751	845	912	966	877	911
Connecticut	814	733	663	710	737	878	811	823	896	838
Delaware	308	278	267	273	272	284	277	358	353	370
D. of Columbia	279	246	231	191	169	188	181	234	246	328
Florida	2,655	2,715	2,504	2,677	3,064	3,496	3,834	4,025	4,285	4,182
Georgia	1,432	1,236	1,206	1,446	1,604	1,848	2,164	2,467	2,681	2,378
Hawaii	133	202	170	250	296	240	276	259	260	362
Idaho	212	228	214	270	291	336	318	325	312	296
Illinois	3,370	2,974	2,822	2,945	3,164	3,266	4,131	4,152	4,240	4,461
Indiana	2,026	1,755	1,734	1,747	1,881	2,034	2,236	2,537	3,232	2,682
Iowa	1,85	1,135	1,173	1,234	1,293	1,483	1,585	1,656	1,746	1,737
Kansas	915	843	812	1,171	1,214	1,191	1,312	1,359	1,403	1,330
Kentucky	1,092	1,148	1,193	1,253	1,424	1,674	1,994	2,190	2,086	1,909
Louisiana	998	999	994	980	1,216	1,201	1,700	1,811	1,847	1,757
Maine	364	288	310	269	326	400	483	594	633	548
Maryland	1,205	1,026	920	1,013	1,107	1,323	1,463	1,665	1,599	1,616
Massachusetts	2,386	2,029	1,685	1,726	1,865	2,016	2,272	2,536	2,604	2,742
Michigan	3,119	2,763	2,701	2,583	2,688	3,016	3,259	3,322	3,321	3,428
Minnesota	1,246	1,125	1,141	1,170	1,385	1,502	1,599	1,664	1,604	1,529
Mississippi	1,035	851	799	911	1,147	1,226	1,369	1,571	1,572	1,605
Missouri	1,461	1,397	1,358	1,456	1,771	1,963	2,175	2,479	2,565	2,532
Montana	245	203	208	225	207	243	215	267	285	241
Nebraska	430	288	321	347	430	613	703	844	927	834
Nevada	153	182	149	153	173	236	228	266	231	297
New Hampshire	311	305	275	313	331	359	503	485	498	502
New Jersey	1,863	1,678	1,570	1,640	1,766	2,027	2,258	2,372	2,319	2,246
New Mexico	430	385	418	550	499	534	566	601	582	603
New York	6,467	6,052	5,712	5,582	5,905	6,867	7,116	7,402	8,232	8,521
North Carolina	1,759	1,722	1,760	2,005	2,342	2,547	2,910	3,063	3,100	2,994
North Dakota	310	179	202	186	215	271	288	294	300	301
Ohio	4,355	3,753	3,459	3,726	3,898	4,350	4,566	4,874	4,964	4,913
Oklahoma	805	786	902	881	1,088	1,181	1,282	1,413	1,349	1,295
Oregon	748	755	643	697	670	776	838	782	795	797
Pennsylvania	4,844	4,459	3,835	4,139	4,315	5,141	5,568	5,763	5,936	5,599
Rhode Island	457	404	393	364	439	430	421	625	624	508
South Carolina	884	846	863	886	1,056	1,096	1,217	1,257	1,254	1,234
South Dakota	324	378	322	365	442	441	414	463	425	403
Tennessee	1,673	1,431	1,296	1,436	1,571	1,936	2,252	2,411	2,632	2,363
Texas	3,347	3,186	3,320	3,951	4,605	5,314	5,720	6,049	5,875	5,564
Utah	402	454	477	475	600	664	644	730	727	702
Vermont	181	145	113	140	153	172	226	222	143	169
Virginia	1,465	1,459	1,356	1,516	1,618	1,913	2,082	2,374	2,314	2,291
Washington	1,293	1,149	1,056	1,185	1,195	1,309	1,287	1,429	1,299	1,302
West Virginia	734	603	614	724	768	776	874	941	863	835
Wisconsin	1,723	1,482	1,219	1,424	1,580	1,770	1,869	2,069	2,138	1,999
Wyoming	118	135	151	191	203	258	274	251	212	220
American Samoa	10	10	10	12	13	12	6	6	7	20
Guam	12	0	0	20	0	0	7	16	11	25
Puerto Rico	1,045	908	962	1,022	989	914	951	915	1,196	1,001
Virgin Islands	12	17	11	6	12	14	10	14	15	19

[1] National and regional totals exclude American Samoa, Guam, Puerto Rico, and the Virgin Islands.

41

Table 29
GRADUATIONS FROM BASIC BACCALAUREATE NURSING PROGRAMS,
BY NLN REGION AND STATE: 1986-87 TO 1995-96[1]

NLN REGION AND STATE	NUMBER OF GRADUATIONS[2]									
	1986-87	1987-88	1988-89	1989-90	1990-91	1991-92	1992-93	1993-94	1994-95	1995-96
United States	23,761	21,504	18,997	18,571	19,264	21,415	24,442	28,912	31,254	32,413
North Atlantic	6,320	5,720	4,802	4,208	4,001	4,294	4,959	5,793	6,556	7,084
Midwest	7,218	6,430	5,756	5,670	5,861	6,523	7,364	8,856	9,746	10,123
South	6,970	6,423	5,804	5,868	6,521	7,570	8,794	10,433	11,033	11,239
West	3,253	2,931	2,635	2,825	2,881	3,028	3,325	3,830	3,919	3,967
Alabama	688	568	511	491	481	522	553	912	1,003	1,017
Alaska	26	26	34	32	21	32	48	46	47	71
Arizona	279	247	230	240	201	186	241	269	317	341
Arkansas	188	200	152	196	185	241	256	297	332	323
California	1,394	1,283	1,163	1,242	1,221	1,184	1,285	1,500	1,515	1,475
Colorado	179	210	179	235	297	364	414	461	419	439
Connecticut	302	286	260	233	214	287	278	292	382	378
Delaware	167	137	105	93	67	90	85	121	161	165
D. of Columbia	218	191	176	146	125	170	155	200	212	283
Florida	561	521	503	513	500	619	724	695	799	905
Georgia	446	415	326	397	453	483	582	777	841	849
Hawaii	89	90	40	72	134	66	96	98	121	157
Idaho	34	26	32	56	71	80	74	73	84	103
Illinois	1,156	984	943	929	841	892	1,019	1,345	1,444	1,634
Indiana	784	774	701	641	632	722	796	975	1,380	1,166
Iowa	410	322	254	231	239	271	304	324	396	406
Kansas	408	291	281	345	386	395	536	590	637	595
Kentucky	319	365	342	331	308	359	464	553	501	526
Louisiana	450	490	505	472	608	601	818	872	937	885
Maine	176	166	159	107	140	165	198	252	270	251
Maryland	379	345	282	262	278	356	390	532	559	609
Massachusetts	862	796	631	598	531	591	684	811	755	903
Michigan	897	850	862	728	753	801	969	933	1,009	1,153
Minnesota	466	415	322	339	389	427	540	578	522	540
Mississippi	359	309	208	250	322	395	425	507	556	522
Missouri	319	352	333	323	333	459	575	710	850	936
Montana	174	144	139	137	100	140	109	152	165	136
Nebraska	152	185	192	227	259	367	391	548	642	578
Nevada	33	35	34	45	61	89	99	98	111	111
New Hampshire	118	97	86	76	81	77	119	120	124	125
New Jersey	413	382	347	318	294	265	339	391	361	432
New Mexico	73	71	50	58	46	59	69	93	93	91
New York	1,959	1,724	1,468	1,227	1,092	1,131	1,305	1,62	1,936	2,096
North Carolina	558	508	440	369	450	586	702	724	779	853
North Dakota	198	179	202	186	215	271	288	294	300	301
Ohio	1,326	1,198	1,006	1,008	1,003	1,012	1,116	1,477	1,458	1,667
Oklahoma	314	254	327	270	316	338	416	439	411	436
Oregon	288	248	221	216	221	270	284	282	314	296
Pennsylvania	1,813	1,677	1,370	1,257	1,289	1,358	1,556	1,697	2,082	2,124
Rhode Island	214	193	154	121	120	123	184	231	224	266
South Carolina	354	309	279	268	277	247	328	375	430	437
South Dakota	157	152	112	121	185	224	117	199	186	199
Tennessee	449	415	336	433	405	552	690	844	1,030	906
Texas	1,232	1,105	1,050	1,076	1,268	1,504	1,697	1,966	1,957	1,984
Utah	192	162	146	146	170	175	188	236	242	248
Vermont	78	71	46	32	48	37	56	50	49	61
Virginia	528	476	426	406	464	541	533	635	588	657
Washington	453	366	333	299	305	332	363	467	439	443
West Virginia	145	143	117	134	206	226	216	305	310	330
Wisconsin	945	728	548	592	626	682	713	883	922	948
Wyoming	39	23	34	47	33	51	55	55	52	56
American Samoa	0	0	0	0	0	0	0	0	0	0
Guam	0	0	0	20	0	0	7	16	11	25
Puerto Rico	553	572	626	569	527	465	412	438	563	464
Virgin Islands	7	9	3	4	6	6	4	5	8	11

[1] National and regional totals exclude American Samoa, Guam, Puerto Rico, and the Virgin Islands.
[2] Includes basic students only.

Table 30
GRADUATIONS FROM ASSOCIATE DEGREE NURSING PROGRAMS,
BY NLN REGION AND STATE: 1986-87 TO 1995-96[1]

NLN REGION AND STATE	NUMBER OF GRADUATIONS									
	1986-87	1987-88	1988-89	1989-90	1990-91	1991-92	1992-93	1993-94	1994-95	1995-96
United States	38,528	37,397	37,837	42,318	46,794	52,896	56,770	58,839	58,749	56,641
North Atlantic	8,530	8,164	8,101	8,778	9,463	11,381	12,040	12,425	12,689	12,489
Midwest	10,418	9,734	10,050	11,234	12,343	13,656	14,767	14,884	15,243	14,579
South	12,794	12,570	12,884	14,851	17,264	19,524	21,656	22,926	22,748	21,286
West	6,786	6,929	6,802	7,455	7,724	8,335	8,307	8,604	8,069	8,287
Alabama	865	842	825	918	1,072	1,307	1,384	1,697	1,840	1,741
Alaska	25	20	30	30	30	45	30	33	27	24
Arizona	516	520	554	567	595	606	677	795	749	716
Arkansas	435	395	400	494	643	731	687	668	636	622
California	3,544	3,519	3,416	3,589	3,652	3,869	3,793	3,915	3,753	3,896
Colorado	342	342	345	349	454	481	498	505	458	472
Connecticut	309	282	227	281	300	405	380	376	346	349
Delaware	129	133	153	172	195	186	184	213	176	186
D. of Columbia	61	55	55	45	44	18	26	34	34	45
Florida	2,017	2,143	1,944	2,098	2,457	2,790	3,037	3,243	3,391	3,277
Georgia	820	745	826	988	1,101	1,365	1,582	1,690	1,840	1,529
Hawaii	44	112	130	178	162	174	180	161	139	205
Idaho	178	202	182	214	220	256	244	252	228	193
Illinois	1,818	1,712	1,724	1,875	2,105	2,281	2,904	2,582	2,614	2,656
Indiana	984	845	952	1,034	1,199	1,289	1,405	1,507	1,767	1,453
Iowa	795	699	807	893	923	1,043	1,038	1,078	1,084	1,091
Kansas	470	519	521	809	808	772	776	769	766	735
Kentucky	773	783	851	922	1,116	1,315	1,530	1,637	1,585	1,383
Louisiana	326	328	295	341	452	574	847	902	875	827
Maine	163	122	151	162	186	235	285	342	363	297
Maryland	732	609	564	653	739	847	942	997	934	914
Massachusetts	1,129	942	890	904	1,048	1,100	1,222	1,346	1,413	1,415
Michigan	2,016	1,755	1,727	1,744	1,802	2,045	2,088	2,164	2,163	2,218
Minnesota	780	710	819	831	996	1,075	1,059	1,086	1,082	989
Mississippi	676	542	591	661	825	831	944	1,064	1,016	1,083
Missouri	677	666	686	775	943	1,100	1,111	1,347	1,325	1,343
Montana	71	59	69	88	107	103	106	115	120	105
Nebraska	56	41	72	80	131	193	255	235	197	199
Nevada	120	147	115	108	112	147	129	168	120	186
New Hampshire	187	179	189	237	250	282	384	365	374	377
New Jersey	975	794	783	904	947	1,139	1,211	1,220	1,200	1,158
New Mexico	357	314	368	492	453	475	497	508	489	512
New York	3,985	4,002	4,025	4,093	4,478	5,365	5,634	5,576	6,102	6,247
North Carolina	1,070	1,126	1,254	1,517	1,695	1,731	1,982	2,110	2,101	1,965
North Dakota	61	0	0	0	0	0	0	0	0	0
Ohio	1,926	1,868	1,896	2,163	2,281	2,585	2,720	2,706	2,838	2,688
Oklahoma	491	532	575	611	772	843	866	974	938	859
Oregon	460	507	422	481	449	506	554	500	481	501
Pennsylvania	1,450	1,412	1,347	1,655	1,607	2,231	2,338	2,417	2,214	2,101
Rhode Island	202	169	214	217	303	285	206	364	373	206
South Carolina	524	537	584	618	779	849	889	882	824	797
South Dakota	139	209	193	224	239	217	297	264	239	204
Tennessee	840	807	824	884	1,014	1,151	1,308	1,256	1,222	1,151
Texas	2,013	1,973	2,161	2,728	3,179	3,605	3,821	3,889	3,710	3,372
Utah	210	292	331	329	430	489	456	494	485	454
Vermont	103	74	67	108	105	135	170	172	94	108
Virginia	709	799	775	909	935	1,105	1,248	1,351	1,355	1,317
Washington	840	783	723	886	890	977	924	962	860	859
West Virginia	503	409	415	509	485	480	589	566	481	449
Wisconsin	696	710	653	806	916	1,056	1,114	1,146	1,168	1,003
Wyoming	79	112	117	144	170	207	219	196	160	164
American Samoa	10	10	10	12	13	12	6	6	7	20
Guam	12	0	0	0	0	0	0	0	0	0
Puerto Rico	492	336	336	453	462	449	539	477	633	537
Virgin Islands	5	8	8	2	6	8	6	9	7	8

[1] National and regional totals exclude American Samoa, Guam, Puerto Rico, and the Virgin Islands.

NLN REGION AND STATE	NUMBER OF GRADUATIONS									
	1986-87	1987-88	1988-89	1989-90	1990-91	1991-92	1992-93	1993-94	1994-95	1995-96
United States	8,272	5,938	4,826	5,199	6,172	6,528	6,937	7,119	7,049	5,703
North Atlantic	3,424	2,733	2,151	2,361	2,814	3,087	3,117	3,196	3,239	2,798
Midwest	3,028	1,908	1,458	1,450	1,757	1,721	2,006	1,973	1,876	1,447
South	1,633	1,130	1,080	1,263	1,429	1,528	1,597	1,774	1,771	1,458
West	187	167	137	125	172	192	217	176	163	0
Alabama	34	20	18	16	12	38	33	33	0	0
Alaska	0	0	0	0	0	0	0	0	0	0
Arizona	0	0	0	0	0	0	0	0	0	0
Arkansas	103	90	135	188	211	252	273	289	284	257
California	187	167	137	125	172	192	217	176	163	0
Colorado	0	0	0	0	0	0	0	0	0	0
Connecticut	203	165	176	196	223	186	153	155	168	111
Delaware	12	8	9	8	10	8	8	24	16	19
D. of Columbia	0	0	0	0	0	0	0	0	0	0
Florida	77	51	57	66	107	87	73	87	95	0
Georgia	166	76	54	61	50	0	0	0	0	0
Hawaii	0	0	0	0	0	0	0	0	0	0
Idaho	0	0	0	0	0	0	0	0	0	0
Illinois	396	278	155	141	218	93	208	225	182	171
Indiana	258	136	81	72	50	23	35	55	85	63
Iowa	180	114	112	110	131	169	243	254	266	240
Kansas	37	33	10	17	20	24	0	0	0	0
Kentucky	0	0	0	0	0	0	0	0	0	0
Louisiana	222	181	194	167	156	26	35	37	35	45
Maine	25	0	0	0	0	0	0	0	0	0
Maryland	94	72	74	98	90	120	131	136	106	93
Massachusetts	395	291	164	224	286	325	366	379	436	424
Michigan	206	158	112	111	133	170	202	225	149	57
Minnesota	0	0	0	0	0	0	0	0	0	0
Mississippi	0	0	0	0	0	0	0	0	0	0
Missouri	465	379	339	358	495	404	489	422	390	253
Montana	0	0	0	0	0	0	0	0	0	0
Nebraska	222	62	57	40	40	53	57	61	88	57
Nevada	0	0	0	0	0	0	0	0	0	0
New Hampshire	14	29	0	0	0	0	0	0	0	0
New Jersey	630	502	440	418	525	623	708	761	758	656
New Mexico	0	0	0	0	0	0	0	0	0	0
New York	523	326	219	262	335	371	177	198	194	178
North Carolina	131	88	66	119	197	230	226	229	220	176
North Dakota	51	0	0	0	0	0	0	0	0	0
Ohio	1,103	687	557	555	614	753	730	691	668	558
Oklahoma	0	0	0	0	0	0	0	0	0	0
Oregon	0	0	0	0	0	0	0	0	0	0
Pennsylvania	1,581	1,370	1,118	1,227	1,419	1,552	1,674	1,649	1,640	1,374
Rhode Island	41	42	25	26	16	22	31	30	27	36
South Carolina	6	0	0	0	0	0	0	0	0	0
South Dakota	28	17	17	20	18	0	0	0	0	0
Tennessee	384	209	136	119	152	233	254	311	380	306
Texas	102	108	109	147	158	205	202	194	208	208
Utah	0	0	0	0	0	0	0	0	0	0
Vermont	0	0	0	0	0	0	0	0	0	0
Virginia	228	184	155	201	219	267	301	388	371	317
Washington	0	0	0	0	0	0	0	0	0	0
West Virginia	86	51	82	81	77	70	69	70	72	56
Wisconsin	82	44	18	26	38	32	42	40	48	48
Wyoming	0	0	0	0	0	0	0	0	0	0
American Samoa	0	0	0	0	0	0	0	0	0	0
Guam	0	0	0	0	0	0	0	0	0	0
Puerto Rico	0	0	0	0	0	0	0	0	0	0
Virgin Islands	0	0	0	0	0	0	0	0	0	0

[1] National and regional totals exclude American Samoa, Guam, Puerto Rico, and the Virgin Islands.

Table 32
BASIC AND RN STUDENT GRADUATIONS FROM BACCALAUREATE NURSING PROGRAMS:
1986-87 TO 1995-96[1]

| YEAR | GRADUATIONS FROM BACCALAUREATE NURSING PROGRAMS | | | |
| | Total Graduations | Basic Programs | | BRN* Programs |
		Basic Students	RN Students	RN Students
1986-87	34,475	23,761	6,591	4,123
1987-88	32,672	21,504	6,710	4,458
1988-89	30,543	18,997	7,195	4,351
1989-90	30,763	18,571	7,241	4,951
1990-91	29,438	19,264	7,027	3,147
1991-92	32,029	21,415	7,064	3,550
1992-93	34,504	24,442	6,360	3,702
1993-94	39,693	28,912	7,018	3,763
1994-95	43,249	31,254	7,296	4,699
1995-96	46,598	32,413	8,288	5,897

[1] Excludes American Samoa, Guam, Puerto Rico, and the Virgin Islands.
* BRN programs are baccalaureate programs that admit only RNs.

Table 33
GRADUATIONS OF REGISTERED NURSES FROM BACCALAUREATE NURSING PROGRAMS,
BY PREVIOUS BASIC NURSING EDUCATION AND REGION: 1991-92 TO 1995-96[1]

| YEAR AND REGION | BACCALAUREATE PROGRAMS ACCEPTING RNs | PREVIOUS NURSING CREDENTIAL[2] | | |
		Total	Diploma	Associate Degree
1991-92 (Total)	637	10,614	3,691	6,923
North Atlantic	158	2,963	1,289	1,674
Midwest	197	3,282	1,298	1,984
South	205	2,926	808	2,118
West	77	1,443	296	1,147
1992-93 (Total)	644	10,062	3,083	6,979
North Atlantic	164	2,741	1,114	1,627
Midwest	201	2,924	1,062	1,862
South	206	2,711	627	2,084
West	73	1,686	280	1,406
1993-94 (Total)	646	10,781	3,792	6,989
North Atlantic	166	3,160	1,377	1,783
Midwest	200	3,133	1,400	1,733
South	207	3,075	760	2,315
West	73	1,413	255	1,158
1994-95 (Total)	665	11,995	3,745	8,250
North Atlantic	168	3,398	1,333	2,065
Midwest	206	3,455	1,194	2,261
South	216	3,403	647	2,756
West	75	1,739	571	1,168
1995-96 (Total)	672	14,185	4,364	9,821
North Atlantic	170	3,786	1,496	2,290
Midwest	208	3,393	1,220	2,173
South	218	3,970	869	3,101
West	76	3,036	779	2,257

[1] Excludes American Samoa, Guam, Puerto Rico, and the Virgin Islands.
[2] Includes RNs in basic programs, RNs in BRN programs, and basic BSN students.

Table 34
TOTAL GRADUATIONS FROM BACCALAUREATE NURSING PROGRAMS, BY NLN REGION AND STATE:
1992 TO 1996[1]

NLN REGION AND STATE	GRADUATIONS FROM BACCALAUREATE NURSING PROGRAMS[2]									
	1992		1993		1994		1995		1996	
	Total	RNs Only	Total	RNs Only	Total	RNs Only	Total	RNs Only	Total	RNs Only
United States	32,029	10,614	34,504	10,062	39,693	10,781	43,249	11,995	46,598	14,185
North Atlantic	7,257	2,963	7,700	2,741	8,953	3,160	9,954	3,398	10,870	3,786
Midwest	9,805	3,282	10,288	2,924	11,989	3,133	13,201	3,455	13,516	3,393
South	10,496	2,926	11,505	2,711	13,508	3,075	14,436	3,403	15,209	3,970
West	4,471	1,443	5,011	1,686	5,243	1,413	5,658	1,739	7,003	3,036
Alabama	773	251	751	198	1,141	229	1,267	264	1,408	391
Alaska	44	12	59	11	51	5	51	4	81	10
Arizona	388	202	546	305	587	318	769	452	1,835	1,494
Arkansas	274	33	297	41	357	60	415	83	380	57
California	1,789	605	1,988	703	1,796	296	2,210	695	2,124	649
Colorado	497	133	614	200	596	135	523	104	642	203
Connecticut	422	135	424	146	464	172	618	236	510	132
Delaware	144	54	181	96	214	93	286	125	301	136
D. of Columbia	216	46	175	20	237	37	236	24	307	24
Florida	1,044	425	1,107	383	1,177	482	1,179	380	1,380	475
Georgia	649	166	756	174	1,003	226	1,141	300	1,191	342
Hawaii	174	108	168	72	157	59	184	63	188	31
Idaho	103	23	130	56	127	54	109	25	171	68
Illinois	1,322	430	1,478	459	1,745	400	1,881	437	2,160	526
Indiana	1,020	298	1,018	222	1,291	316	1,742	362	1,560	394
Iowa	461	190	443	139	481	157	609	213	570	164
Kansas	521	126	639	103	705	115	705	68	700	105
Kentucky	541	182	581	117	658	105	639	138	686	160
Louisiana	692	91	898	80	960	88	1,031	94	991	106
Maine	201	36	230	32	288	36	323	53	320	69
Maryland	671	315	664	274	795	263	747	188	821	212
Massachusetts	961	370	988	304	1,203	392	1,141	386	1,315	412
Michigan	1,357	556	1,537	568	1,412	479	1,646	637	1,564	411
Minnesota	599	172	710	170	831	253	712	190	723	183
Mississippi	455	60	502	77	574	67	660	104	662	140
Missouri	812	353	921	346	1,157	447	1,365	515	1,463	527
Montana	154	14	120	11	164	12	179	14	147	11
Nebraska	525	158	490	99	643	95	746	104	696	118
Nevada	104	15	116	17	117	19	133	22	121	10
New Hampshire	111	34	176	57	184	64	208	84	231	106
New Jersey	515	250	572	233	664	273	641	280	799	367
New Mexico	119	60	149	80	184	91	199	106	190	99
New York	2,164	1,033	2,372	1,067	2,687	1,059	3,163	1,227	3,345	1,249
North Carolina	865	279	988	286	1,088	364	1,094	315	1,217	364
North Dakota	305	34	334	46	354	60	346	46	359	58
Ohio	1,603	591	1,636	520	2,050	573	2,030	572	2,326	659
Oklahoma	427	89	499	83	498	59	491	80	517	81
Oregon	328	58	295	11	345	63	385	71	381	85
Pennsylvania	2,289	931	2,268	712	2,605	908	2,974	892	3,328	1,204
Rhode Island	170	47	234	50	324	93	263	39	306	40
South Carolina	324	77	452	124	476	101	545	115	564	127
South Dakota	293	69	174	57	252	53	249	63	257	58
Tennessee	801	249	934	244	1,067	223	1,304	274	1,279	373
Texas	1,889	385	2,051	354	2,401	435	2,413	456	2,424	440
Utah	247	72	262	74	345	109	332	90	375	127
Vermont	64	27	80	24	83	33	101	52	108	47
Virginia	789	248	758	225	914	279	1,018	430	1,269	612
Washington	454	122	505	142	716	249	528	89	674	231
West Virginia	302	76	267	51	399	94	492	182	420	90
Wisconsin	987	305	908	195	1,068	185	1,170	248	1,138	190
Wyoming	70	19	59	4	58	3	56	4	74	18
American Samoa	0	0	0	0	0	0	0	0	0	0
Guam	0	0	14	7	16	0	14	3	25	0
Puerto Rico	598	133	620	208	572	134	642	79	553	89
Virgin Islands	7	1	6	2	11	6	9	1	12	1

[1] National and regional totals exclude American Samoa, Guam, Puerto Rico, and the Virgin Islands.
[2] Totals include RNs in basic programs, RNs in BRN programs, and basic BSN students.

Table 35
APPLICATIONS PER FALL ADMISSION
FOR BASIC RN PROGRAMS, BY TYPE
OF PROGRAM AND NLN REGION: 1996

NLN REGION[1]	NUMBER OF APPLICATIONS	NUMBER OF FALL ADMISSIONS	APPLICATIONS PER FALL ADMISSIONS
ALL REPORTING RN PROGRAMS[2]			
All Regions	172,749	71,049	2.43
N. Atlantic	44,516	17,161	2.59
Midwest	41,878	18,695	2.24
South	63,644	26,726	2.38
West	22,711	8,467	2.68
BACCALAUREATE PROGRAMS			
All Regions	60,784	24,254	2.51
N. Atlantic	15,875	5,389	2.95
Midwest	16,396	6,941	2.36
South	21,234	9,092	2.34
West	7,279	2,832	2.57
ASSOCIATE DEGREE PROGRAMS			
All Regions	102,748	42,817	2.40
N. Atlantic	23,664	9,776	2.42
Midwest	23,210	10,755	2.16
South	40,442	16,651	2.43
West	15,432	5,635	2.74
DIPLOMA PROGRAMS			
All Regions	9,217	3,978	2.32
N. Atlantic	4,977	1,996	2.49
Midwest	2,272	999	2.27
South	1,968	983	2.00
West	0	0	0

[1] Excludes American Samoa, Guam, Puerto Rico and the Virgin Islands.

[2] To be included in this tabulation, a nursing program must have answered the question on number of applications and must have admitted a class in the fall of the survey year.

Table 36
PERCENTAGE OF APPLICATIONS FOR ADMISSION
ACCEPTED AND NOT ACCEPTED AND PERCENTAGE ON
WAITING LISTS FOR ALL BASIC RN PROGRAMS, BY
TYPE OF PROGRAM: 1996

ALL REPORTING RN PROGRAMS	
Total applications	100.0
Accepted	51.5
Not accepted	48.5
Percent of qualified applicants not accepted and placed on waiting lists.	12.3
BACCALAUREATE PROGRAMS	
Total applications	100.0
Accepted	55.1
Not accepted	44.9
Percent of qualified applicants not accepted and placed on waiting lists.	6.4
ASSOCIATE DEGREE PROGRAMS	
Total applications	100.0
Accepted	48.3
Not accepted	51.7
Percent of qualified applicants not accepted and placed on waiting lists.	16.6
DIPLOMA PROGRAMS	
Total applications	100.0
Accepted	61.0
Not accepted	39.0
Percent of qualified applicants not accepted and placed on waiting lists.	4.7

Section 4
Numeric Tables
on Male and Minority Students

Table 1
ESTIMATED NUMBER OF STUDENT ADMISSIONS
TO ALL BASIC RN PROGRAMS, BY RACE/ETHNICITY, NLN REGION AND STATE: 1995–1996*

NLN REGION AND STATE	NUMBER OF PROGRAMS	TOTAL** NUMBER OF ADMISSIONS	NUMBER OF ADMISSIONS				
			White	Black	Hispanic	Asian	American Indian
United States	1,508	119,205	96,416	12,123	4,715	5,017	901
North Atlantic	327	29,600	22,820	4,277	1,113	1,232	154
Midwest	442	32,060	28,702	1,753	528	915	149
South	514	42,945	34,352	5,526	1,778	945	339
West	225	14,600	10,542	567	1,296	1,925	259
Alabama	36	3,438	2,645	708	19	44	22
Alaska	2	111	93	4	6	3	5
Arizona	17	1,415	1,207	30	108	46	23
Arkansas	22	1,398	1,203	153	9	17	16
California	95	6,814	4,037	421	813	1,447	92
Colorado	16	931	793	41	75	15	5
Connecticut	16	1,095	936	95	33	30	1
Delaware	7	422	320	86	5	9	2
D. of Columbia	5	335	207	78	15	30	5
Florida	39	5,094	3,784	740	388	155	26
Georgia	33	2,890	2,383	411	36	53	6
Hawaii	7	381	172	6	14	189	0
Idaho	7	341	312	1	9	13	5
Illinois	73	5,852	4,549	605	228	455	20
Indiana	46	3,595	3,349	151	42	39	12
Iowa	42	2,087	2,024	22	17	19	3
Kansas	29	1,426	1,291	80	21	24	7
Kentucky	34	2,421	2,313	65	12	16	15
Louisiana	23	2,193	1,755	391	24	18	5
Maine	15	655	634	5	3	7	5
Maryland	23	2,138	1,579	425	25	97	12
Massachusetts	44	3,337	2,819	288	136	92	2
Michigan	48	3,943	3,600	143	78	97	22
Minnesota	24	1,882	1,718	71	16	60	17
Mississippi	23	2,155	1,780	349	8	12	5
Missouri	50	3,316	2,990	236	21	57	11
Montana	5	359	315	4	5	3	31
Nebraska	14	870	816	15	13	24	2
Nevada	6	322	282	8	7	22	4
New Hampshire	9	595	575	8	4	5	3
New Jersey	37	3,080	1,994	618	192	236	40
New Mexico	15	704	492	13	149	8	40
New York	101	12,997	9,069	2,602	613	633	79
North Carolina	62	3,919	3,384	412	31	64	31
North Dakota	7	382	361	0	1	4	16
Ohio	67	5,814	5,291	359	59	89	12
Oklahoma	28	1,629	1,316	92	30	47	146
Oregon	16	850	763	5	12	49	19
Pennsylvania	82	6,335	5,623	452	85	159	14
Rhode Island	7	568	467	44	27	27	3
South Carolina	21	1,752	1,452	262	12	23	2
South Dakota	10	417	393	4	1	2	16
Tennessee	36	2,950	2,610	273	25	34	6
Texas	77	7,093	4,878	771	1,126	274	40
Utah	7	590	536	1	31	15	7
Vermont	4	181	176	1	0	4	0
Virginia	37	2,807	2,230	453	32	89	3
Washington	24	1,550	1,322	32	59	113	25
West Virginia	20	1,068	1,040	21	1	2	4
Wisconsin	32	2,476	2,320	67	31	45	11
Wyoming	8	232	218	1	8	2	3

*Excludes American Samoa, Guam, Puerto Rico and the Virgin Islands.
**Due to rounding, the racial/ethnic estimations sometimes add up to slightly more or less than the true total.

Table 2
ESTIMATED NUMBER OF STUDENT ADMISSIONS TO BASIC BACCALAUREATE
NURSING PROGRAMS, BY RACE/ETHNICITY, NLN REGION AND STATE: 1995-1996*

NLN REGION AND STATE	NUMBER OF PROGRAMS	TOTAL** NUMBER OF ADMISSIONS	NUMBER OF ADMISSIONS				
			White	Black	Hispanic	Asian	American Indian
United States	523	40,048	32,095	3,736	1,676	2,289	244
North Atlantic	117	9,240	7,388	1,002	297	527	28
Midwest	164	11,922	10,512	635	227	501	44
South	181	13,995	10,733	1,966	775	423	96
West	61	4,891	3,462	133	377	838	76
Alabama	13	1,101	855	214	9	20	3
Alaska	1	79	65	3	5	3	3
Arizona	4	471	383	11	42	22	12
Arkansas	9	429	369	40	7	9	4
California	24	1,872	1,025	79	203	540	24
Colorado	7	415	361	15	26	10	3
Connecticut	8	503	447	32	10	14	0
Delaware	2	174	108	57	1	7	1
D. of Columbia	4	275	207	28	10	25	5
Florida	13	1,020	657	155	162	42	3
Georgia	14	980	785	150	13	31	0
Hawaii	3	191	43	6	6	137	0
Idaho	3	130	112	0	3	11	3
Illinois	27	2,102	1,600	189	90	224	2
Indiana	20	1,474	1,373	60	22	17	2
Iowa	12	509	493	2	4	7	2
Kansas	11	577	523	24	7	17	5
Kentucky	10	690	648	27	4	10	1
Louisiana	13	1,216	894	293	17	11	1
Maine	7	294	282	0	2	6	4
Maryland	7	728	517	152	15	38	6
Massachusetts	16	1,174	1,039	61	35	41	0
Michigan	15	1,255	1,069	80	37	61	8
Minnesota	9	697	650	8	5	32	1
Mississippi	7	568	453	103	3	7	3
Missouri	17	1,364	1,203	107	16	35	3
Montana	2	225	208	4	4	3	5
Nebraska	6	541	504	6	7	23	1
Nevada	2	125	105	4	3	13	0
New Hampshire	3	171	168	1	1	1	0
New Jersey	9	472	309	72	32	56	3
New Mexico	2	193	137	2	44	4	6
New York	33	3,021	2,075	529	153	253	11
North Carolina	12	1,123	938	139	8	32	7
North Dakota	7	382	361	0	1	4	16
Ohio	22	1,771	1,593	112	15	47	2
Oklahoma	11	544	430	37	12	25	42
Oregon	3	337	282	3	8	35	7
Pennsylvania	31	2,838	2,479	208	41	107	3
Rhode Island	3	246	205	13	12	15	1
South Carolina	8	429	338	80	4	5	2
South Dakota	4	179	173	2	1	2	1
Tennessee	18	1,320	1,214	73	12	15	5
Texas	25	2,693	1,735	299	499	138	19
Utah	3	262	235	1	14	9	3
Vermont	1	72	69	1	0	2	0
Virginia	12	755	514	193	9	39	0
Washington	6	543	467	4	13	50	9
West Virginia	9	399	386	11	1	1	0
Wisconsin	14	1,071	970	45	22	32	1
Wyoming	1	48	39	1	6	1	1

*Excludes American Samoa, Guam, Puerto Rico, and the Virgin Islands.
**Due to rounding, the racial/ethnic estimations sometimes add up to slightly more or less than the true total.

Table 3
ESTIMATED NUMBER OF STUDENT ADMISSIONS TO ASSOCIATE DEGREE
NURSING PROGRAMS, BY RACE/ETHNICITY, NLN REGION AND STATE: 1995-1996*

NLN REGION AND STATE	NUMBER OF PROGRAMS	TOTAL** NUMBER OF ADMISSIONS	NUMBER OF ADMISSIONS				
			White	Black	Hispanic	Asian	American Indian
United States	876	72,930	59,251	7,697	2,830	2,488	640
North Atlantic	152	16,930	12,771	2,814	682	539	119
Midwest	250	18,746	16,960	1,037	277	363	99
South	310	27,545	22,440	3,412	952	499	239
West	164	9,709	7,080	434	919	1,087	183
Alabama	23	2,337	1,790	494	10	24	19
Alaska	1	32	28	1	1	0	2
Arizona	13	944	824	19	66	24	11
Arkansas	11	734	639	77	1	6	11
California	71	4,942	3,012	342	610	907	68
Colorado	9	516	432	26	49	5	2
Connecticut	6	470	386	52	17	14	1
Delaware	4	218	185	27	4	1	1
D. of Columbia	1	60	0	50	5	5	0
Florida	26	4,074	3,127	585	226	113	23
Georgia	19	1,910	1,598	261	23	22	6
Hawaii	4	190	129	0	8	52	0
Idaho	4	211	200	1	6	2	2
Illinois	42	3,534	2,797	410	121	193	15
Indiana	25	2,061	1,923	84	20	22	10
Iowa	25	1,492	1,452	17	12	9	1
Kansas	18	849	768	56	14	7	2
Kentucky	24	1,731	1,665	38	8	6	14
Louisiana	9	938	822	98	7	7	4
Maine	8	361	352	5	1	1	1
Maryland	14	1,324	987	263	10	58	6
Massachusetts	21	1,751	1,447	180	88	34	1
Michigan	31	2,636	2,481	63	40	35	14
Minnesota	15	1,185	1,068	63	11	28	16
Mississippi	16	1,587	1,327	246	5	5	2
Missouri	30	1,731	1,584	114	5	19	8
Montana	3	134	107	0	1	0	26
Nebraska	7	244	231	8	4	1	0
Nevada	4	197	177	4	4	9	4
New Hampshire	6	424	407	7	3	4	3
New Jersey	14	1,412	933	302	74	67	36
New Mexico	13	511	355	11	105	4	34
New York	63	9,767	6,815	2,061	451	372	67
North Carolina	47	2,570	2,243	260	20	27	22
North Dakota	0	0	0	0	0	0	0
Ohio	34	3,371	3,086	198	41	36	8
Oklahoma	17	1,085	886	55	18	22	104
Oregon	13	513	481	2	4	14	12
Pennsylvania	23	2,068	1,908	100	24	27	7
Rhode Island	3	290	231	30	15	12	2
South Carolina	13	1,323	1,114	182	8	18	0
South Dakota	6	238	220	2	0	0	15
Tennessee	14	1,371	1,184	155	12	18	1
Texas	50	4,204	3,000	465	587	130	21
Utah	4	328	301	0	17	6	4
Vermont	3	109	107	0	0	2	0
Virginia	17	1,688	1,404	223	17	42	2
Washington	18	1,007	855	28	46	63	16
West Virginia	10	669	654	10	0	1	4
Wisconsin	17	1,405	1,350	22	9	13	10
Wyoming	7	184	179	0	2	1	2

*Excludes American Samoa, Guam, Puerto Rico, and the Virgin Islands.
**Due to rounding, the racial/ethnic estimations sometimes add up to slightly more or less
 than the true total

Table 4
ESTIMATED NUMBER OF STUDENT ADMISSIONS TO DIPLOMA
NURSING PROGRAMS, BY RACE/ETHNICITY, NLN REGION AND STATE: 1995-1996*

NLN REGION AND STATE	NUMBER OF PROGRAMS	TOTAL** NUMBER OF ADMISSIONS	NUMBER OF ADMISSIONS				
			White	Black	Hispanic	Asian	American Indian
United States	109	6,227	5,070	690	209	240	17
North Atlantic	58	3,430	2,661	461	134	166	7
Midwest	28	1,392	1,230	81	24	51	6
South	23	1,405	1,179	148	51	23	4
West	0	0	0	0	0	0	0
Alabama	0	0	0	0	0	0	0
Alaska	0	0	0	0	0	0	0
Arizona	0	0	0	0	0	0	0
Arkansas	2	235	195	36	1	2	1
California	0	0	0	0	0	0	0
Colorado	0	0	0	0	0	0	0
Connecticut	2	122	103	11	6	2	0
Delaware	1	30	27	2	0	1	0
D. of Columbia	0	0	0	0	0	0	0
Florida	0	0	0	0	0	0	0
Georgia	0	0	0	0	0	0	0
Hawaii	0	0	0	0	0	0	0
Idaho	0	0	0	0	0	0	0
Illinois	4	216	152	6	17	38	3
Indiana	1	60	53	7	0	0	0
Iowa	5	86	79	3	1	3	0
Kansas	0	0	0	0	0	0	0
Kentucky	0	0	0	0	0	0	0
Louisiana	1	39	39	0	0	0	0
Maine	0	0	0	0	0	0	0
Maryland	2	86	75	10	0	1	0
Massachusetts	7	412	333	47	13	17	1
Michigan	2	52	50	0	1	1	0
Minnesota	0	0	0	0	0	0	0
Mississippi	0	0	0	0	0	0	0
Missouri	3	221	203	15	0	3	0
Montana	0	0	0	0	0	0	0
Nebraska	1	85	81	1	2	0	1
Nevada	0	0	0	0	0	0	0
New Hampshire	0	0	0	0	0	0	0
New Jersey	14	1,196	752	244	86	113	1
New Mexico	0	0	0	0	0	0	0
New York	5	209	179	12	9	8	1
North Carolina	3	226	203	13	3	5	2
North Dakota	0	0	0	0	0	0	0
Ohio	11	672	612	49	3	6	2
Oklahoma	0	0	0	0	0	0	0
Oregon	0	0	0	0	0	0	0
Pennsylvania	28	1,429	1,236	144	20	25	4
Rhode Island	1	32	31	1	0	0	0
South Carolina	0	0	0	0	0	0	0
South Dakota	0	0	0	0	0	0	0
Tennessee	4	259	212	45	1	1	0
Texas	2	196	143	7	40	6	0
Utah	0	0	0	0	0	0	0
Vermont	0	0	0	0	0	0	0
Virginia	8	364	312	37	6	8	1
Washington	0	0	0	0	0	0	0
West Virginia	1	0	0	0	0	0	0
Wisconsin	1	0	0	0	0	0	0
Wyoming	0	0	0	0	0	0	0

*Excludes American Samoa, Guam, Puerto Rico, and the Virgin Islands.
**Due to rounding, the racial/ethnic estimations sometimes add up to slightly more or less than the true total.

Table 5
TRENDS IN THE ESTIMATED NUMBER OF ANNUAL ADMISSIONS
OF MINORITY STUDENTS TO BASIC RN PROGRAMS, 1990-91 TO 1995-96[1]

YEAR	BLACK		HISPANIC		ASIAN		AMERICAN INDIAN	
	Number	Percent	Number	Percent	Number	Percent	Number	Percent
ALL REPORTING RN PROGRAMS								
1990-91	10,822	9.5	3,619	3.2	3,536	3.1	840	0.7
1991-92	10,476	8.5	4,258	3.5	3,972	3.2	874	0.7
1992-93	11,064	8.7	3,834	3.0	4,144	3.3	812	0.6
1993-94	11,514	8.9	4,186	3.2	4,462	3.4	959	0.7
1994-95	11,779	9.3	4,518	3.5	5,285	4.2	997	0.8
1995-96	12,123	10.2	4,715	4.0	5,017	4.2	901	0.7
BACCALAUREATE PROGRAMS								
1990-91	3,363	10.0	1,053	3.1	1,336	4.0	265	0.8
1991-92	3,273	8.6	1,490	3.9	1,531	4.0	283	0.7
1992-93	4,011	9.7	1,079	2.6	1,664	4.0	211	0.5
1993-94	4,005	9.3	1,312	3.0	1,738	4.0	241	0.6
1994-95	3,780	8.7	1,600	3.7	·2,376	5.5	271	0.6
1995-96	3,736	9.3	1,676	4.2	2,289	5.7	244	0.6
ASSOCIATE DEGREE PROGRAMS								
1990-91	6,521	9.3	2,327	3.3	1,920	2.7	552	0.8
1991-92	6,413	8.7	2,459	3.3	2,142	2.9	568	0.8
1992-93	6,406	8.5	2,509	3.3	2,159	2.9	575	0.8
1993-94	6,867	8.9	2,645	3.4	2,461	3.2	691	0.9
1994-95	7,487	9.8	2,671	3.5	2,666	3.5	700	0.9
1995-96	7,697	10.5	2,830	3.9	2,488	3.4	640	0.9
DIPLOMA PROGRAMS								
1990-91	937	9.2	239	2.3	285	2.8	24	0.2
1991-92	790	7.4	309	2.9	299	2.8	23	0.2
1992-93	647	6.4	246	2.4	321	3.2	26	0.3
1993-94	642	6.7	229	2.4	263	2.7	27	0.3
1994-95	512	6.6	247	3.2	243	3.1	26	0.3
1995-96	690	11.1	209	3.4	240	3.8	17	0.3

[1] Excludes American Samoa, Guam, Puerto Rico, and the Virgin Islands.

Table 6
ESTIMATED NUMBER OF STUDENT ENROLLMENTS IN ALL BASIC
RN PROGRAMS, BY RACE/ETHNICITY, NLN REGION AND STATE: 1996*

NLN REGION AND STATE	NUMBER OF PROGRAMS	TOTAL** NUMBER OF ENROLLMENTS	NUMBER OF ENROLLMENTS				
			White	Black	Hispanic	Asian	American Indian
United States	1,508	238,244	193,050	23,611	9,227	10,529	1,816
North Atlantic	327	63,043	49,974	7,833	2,285	2,660	280
Midwest	442	63,041	56,493	3,201	1,183	1,803	356
South	514	83,674	66,479	11,432	3,157	1,938	669
West	225	28,486	20,104	1,145	2,602	4,128	511
Alabama	36	6,713	5,127	1,426	51	82	25
Alaska	2	265	220	12	11	10	12
Arizona	17	2,363	2,050	40	168	66	39
Arkansas	22	2,650	2,331	255	20	26	18
California	95	13,242	7,596	829	1,684	2,965	168
Colorado	16	1,780	1,516	47	157	39	24
Connecticut	16	2,481	2,103	191	99	86	2
Delaware	7	1,117	995	73	16	27	5
D. of Columbia	5	908	650	138	36	76	6
Florida	39	8,453	6,421	995	639	357	39
Georgia	33	5,011	4,108	730	58	101	16
Hawaii	7	1,067	393	44	16	610	7
Idaho	7	700	657	2	13	19	9
Illinois	73	11,231	9,010	843	451	887	38
Indiana	46	6,216	5,797	235	116	49	19
Iowa	42	3,464	3,361	41	23	29	7
Kansas	29	2,840	2,576	142	50	47	26
Kentucky	34	4,584	4,368	137	26	42	13
Louisiana	23	8,830	6,247	2,323	122	92	46
Maine	15	1,774	1,731	7	5	13	19
Maryland	23	3,811	2,754	826	56	154	20
Massachusetts	44	7,549	6,338	731	231	239	8
Michigan	48	8,070	7,268	382	169	188	63
Minnesota	24	3,130	2,895	106	32	70	27
Mississippi	23	3,543	3,029	481	9	18	4
Missouri	50	5,618	5,039	422	36	105	14
Montana	5	858	761	11	16	12	58
Nebraska	14	2,127	1,963	54	48	53	11
Nevada	6	634	535	14	35	39	11
New Hampshire	9	1,246	1,211	15	7	10	3
New Jersey	37	6,212	4,167	1,114	388	523	21
New Mexico	15	1,272	826	28	296	24	98
New York	101	26,101	18,741	4,637	1,268	1,266	183
North Carolina	62	6,894	5,767	879	72	108	69
North Dakota	7	707	661	3	4	5	34
Ohio	67	12,494	11,308	762	134	251	38
Oklahoma	28	3,002	2,433	138	66	72	294
Oregon	16	1,683	1,495	18	39	100	31
Pennsylvania	82	13,820	12,409	856	175	352	26
Rhode Island	7	1,414	1,218	69	60	60	7
South Carolina	21	3,592	2,946	558	32	50	5
South Dakota	10	1,060	991	9	4	8	47
Tennessee	36	5,758	5,110	522	46	68	12
Texas	77	12,742	8,904	1,321	1,884	549	87
Utah	7	1,248	1,155	4	56	21	12
Vermont	4	421	411	2	0	8	0
Virginia	37	5,821	4,713	812	69	215	13
Washington	24	2,947	2,503	94	91	220	38
West Virginia	20	2,270	2,221	29	7	4	8
Wisconsin	32	6,084	5,624	202	116	111	32
Wyoming	8	427	397	2	20	3	4

*Excludes American Samoa, Guam, Puerto Rico and the Virgin Islands.
**Due to rounding, the racial/ethnic estimations sometimes add up to slightly more or less than the true total.

Table 7
ESTIMATED NUMBER OF STUDENT ENROLLMENTS IN BASIC BACCALAUREATE
NURSING PROGRAMS, BY RACE/ETHNICITY, NLN REGION AND STATE: 1996*

NLN REGION AND STATE	NUMBER OF PROGRAMS	TOTAL** NUMBER OF ENROLLMENTS	NUMBER OF ENROLLMENTS				
			White	Black	Hispanic	Asian	American Indian
United States	523	103,213	81,979	10,648	3,990	5,925	676
North Atlantic	117	25,064	20,134	2,590	889	1,378	67
Midwest	164	30,910	27,164	1,684	709	1,201	158
South	181	35,279	26,508	6,013	1,398	1,115	246
West	61	11,960	8,173	361	994	2,231	205
Alabama	13	3,193	2,328	752	36	60	17
Alaska	1	207	170	10	9	9	9
Arizona	4	866	724	12	69	35	26
Arkansas	9	886	794	65	9	15	3
California	24	4,916	2,656	237	565	1,403	55
Colorado	7	981	827	15	94	25	23
Connecticut	8	1,421	1,268	66	28	58	1
Delaware	2	652	585	33	7	25	1
D. of Columbia	4	833	645	78	31	71	6
Florida	13	2,304	1,555	273	300	166	9
Georgia	14	2,208	1,812	306	19	72	0
Hawaii	3	762	240	18	16	482	7
Idaho	3	287	258	0	7	13	9
Illinois	27	5,460	4,179	464	265	540	13
Indiana	20	3,023	2,834	104	51	28	6
Iowa	12	1,266	1,218	15	10	20	3
Kansas	11	1,484	1,329	70	32	35	20
Kentucky	10	1,741	1,611	83	16	30	1
Louisiana	13	6,501	4,290	2,025	80	77	29
Maine	7	1,174	1,143	0	4	10	17
Maryland	7	1,579	1,115	352	26	79	7
Massachusetts	16	3,825	3,264	291	96	170	4
Michigan	15	3,838	3,297	256	114	133	38
Minnesota	9	1,153	1,086	12	11	41	3
Mississippi	7	1,020	890	119	5	6	0
Missouri	17	2,923	2,561	268	23	68	4
Montana	2	640	582	11	14	12	21
Nebraska	6	1,521	1,389	42	43	43	6
Nevada	2	290	229	10	27	23	1
New Hampshire	3	500	490	2	3	5	0
New Jersey	9	1,472	869	265	136	202	0
New Mexico	2	432	284	10	110	13	15
New York	33	7,299	4,823	1,417	468	560	29
North Carolina	12	2,010	1,479	450	20	50	11
North Dakota	7	707	661	3	4	5	34
Ohio	22	5,342	4,772	314	60	185	10
Oklahoma	11	1,133	863	72	27	48	123
Oregon	3	717	607	8	19	70	13
Pennsylvania	31	6,752	6,030	411	76	229	5
Rhode Island	3	893	782	25	40	42	4
South Carolina	8	1,556	1,239	272	12	31	2
South Dakota	4	563	546	5	3	5	4
Tennessee	18	2,592	2,338	186	19	38	11
Texas	25	5,173	3,426	607	796	317	28
Utah	3	576	533	4	21	12	6
Vermont	1	243	235	2	0	6	0
Virginia	12	2,254	1,665	434	29	122	5
Washington	6	1,191	982	25	32	133	19
West Virginia	9	1,129	1,103	17	4	4	0
Wisconsin	14	3,630	3,292	131	93	98	17
Wyoming	1	95	81	1	11	1	1

*Excludes American Samoa, Guam, Puerto Rico, and the Virgin Islands.
**Due to rounding, the racial/ethnic estimations sometimes add up to slightly more or less than the true total.

Table 8
ESTIMATED NUMBER OF STUDENT ENROLLMENTS IN ASSOCIATE DEGREE
NURSING PROGRAMS, BY RACE/ETHNICITY, NLN REGION AND STATE: 1996*

NLN REGION AND STATE	NUMBER OF PROGRAMS	TOTAL** NUMBER OF ENROLLMENTS	NUMBER OF ENROLLMENTS				
			White	Black	Hispanic	Asian	American Indian
United States	876	122,242	100,193	11,838	4,882	4,206	1,109
North Atlantic	152	31,059	24,146	4,568	1,165	980	198
Midwest	250	29,135	26,605	1,349	438	544	187
South	310	45,522	37,511	5,137	1,671	785	418
West	164	16,526	11,931	784	1,608	1,897	306
Alabama	23	3,520	2,799	674	15	22	8
Alaska	1	58	50	2	2	1	3
Arizona	13	1,497	1,326	28	99	31	13
Arkansas	11	1,237	1,089	121	8	6	13
California	71	8,326	4,940	592	1,119	1,562	113
Colorado	9	799	689	32	63	14	1
Connecticut	6	890	703	104	60	23	0
Delaware	4	399	356	34	6	1	2
D. of Columbia	1	75	5	60	5	5	0
Florida	26	6,149	4,866	722	339	191	30
Georgia	19	2,803	2,296	424	39	29	16
Hawaii	4	305	153	26	0	128	0
Idaho	4	413	399	2	6	6	0
Illinois	42	5,255	4,393	353	169	317	20
Indiana	25	3,039	2,822	121	63	20	13
Iowa	25	1,864	1,824	19	10	4	4
Kansas	18	1,356	1,247	72	18	12	6
Kentucky	24	2,843	2,757	54	10	12	12
Louisiana	9	2,264	1,894	296	42	15	17
Maine	8	600	588	7	1	3	2
Maryland	14	2,072	1,495	461	29	73	13
Massachusetts	21	2,840	2,303	373	110	51	2
Michigan	31	4,139	3,882	124	53	55	25
Minnesota	15	1,977	1,809	94	21	29	24
Mississippi	16	2,523	2,139	362	4	12	4
Missouri	30	2,365	2,169	138	13	32	10
Montana	3	218	179	0	2	0	37
Nebraska	7	479	450	12	4	9	4
Nevada	4	344	306	4	8	16	10
New Hampshire	6	746	721	13	4	5	3
New Jersey	14	2,429	1,641	519	122	128	21
New Mexico	13	840	542	18	186	11	83
New York	63	18,479	13,637	3,205	788	693	152
North Carolina	47	4,427	3,882	392	44	53	57
North Dakota	0	0	0	0	0	0	0
Ohio	34	5,767	5,283	343	63	52	25
Oklahoma	17	1,869	1,570	66	39	24	171
Oregon	13	966	888	10	20	30	18
Pennsylvania	23	4,007	3,682	211	49	52	13
Rhode Island	3	416	334	42	20	17	3
South Carolina	13	2,036	1,707	286	20	19	3
South Dakota	6	497	445	4	1	3	43
Tennessee	14	2,655	2,330	270	26	28	1
Texas	50	7,231	5,221	706	1,022	225	59
Utah	4	672	622	0	35	9	6
Vermont	3	178	176	0	0	2	0
Virginia	17	2,756	2,352	291	31	76	6
Washington	18	1,756	1,521	69	59	87	19
West Virginia	10	1,137	1,114	12	3	0	8
Wisconsin	17	2,397	2,281	69	23	11	13
Wyoming	7	332	316	1	9	2	3

*Excludes American Samoa, Guam, Puerto Rico, and the Virgin Islands.
**Due to rounding, the racial/ethnic estimations sometimes add up to slightly more or less than the true total.

Table 9
ESTIMATED NUMBER OF STUDENT ENROLLMENTS IN DIPLOMA
NURSING PROGRAMS, BY RACE/ETHNICITY, NLN REGION AND STATE: 1996*

NLN REGION AND STATE	NUMBER OF PROGRAMS	TOTAL** NUMBER OF ENROLLMENTS	NUMBER OF ENROLLMENTS				
			White	Black	Hispanic	Asian	American Indian
United States	109	12,789	10,878	1,125	355	398	31
North Atlantic	58	6,920	5,694	675	231	302	15
Midwest	28	2,996	2,724	168	36	58	11
South	23	2,873	2,460	282	88	38	5
West	0	0	0	0	0	0	0
Alabama	0	0	0	0	0	0	0
Alaska	0	0	0	0	0	0	0
Arizona	0	0	0	0	0	0	0
Arkansas	2	527	448	69	3	5	2
California	0	0	0	0	0	0	0
Colorado	0	0	0	0	0	0	0
Connecticut	2	170	132	21	11	5	1
Delaware	1	66	54	6	3	1	2
D. of Columbia	0	0	0	0	0	0	0
Florida	0	0	0	0	0	0	0
Georgia	0	0	0	0	0	0	0
Hawaii	0	0	0	0	0	0	0
Idaho	0	0	0	0	0	0	0
Illinois	4	516	438	26	17	30	5
Indiana	1	154	141	10	2	1	0
Iowa	5	334	319	7	3	5	0
Kansas	0	0	0	0	0	0	0
Kentucky	0	0	0	0	0	0	0
Louisiana	1	65	63	2	0	0	0
Maine	0	0	0	0	0	0	0
Maryland	2	160	144	13	1	2	0
Massachusetts	7	884	771	67	25	18	2
Michigan	2	93	89	2	2	0	0
Minnesota	0	0	0	0	0	0	0
Mississippi	0	0	0	0	0	0	0
Missouri	3	330	309	16	0	5	0
Montana	0	0	0	0	0	0	0
Nebraska	1	127	124	0	1	1	1
Nevada	0	0	0	0	0	0	0
New Hampshire	0	0	0	0	0	0	0
New Jersey	14	2,311	1,657	330	130	193	0
New Mexico	0	0	0	0	0	0	0
New York	5	323	281	15	12	13	2
North Carolina	3	457	406	37	8	5	1
North Dakota	0	0	0	0	0	0	0
Ohio	11	1,385	1,253	105	11	14	3
Oklahoma	0	0	0	0	0	0	0
Oregon	0	0	0	0	0	0	0
Pennsylvania	28	3,061	2,697	234	50	71	8
Rhode Island	1	105	102	2	0	1	0
South Carolina	0	0	0	0	0	0	0
South Dakota	0	0	0	0	0	0	0
Tennessee	4	511	442	66	1	2	0
Texas	2	338	257	8	66	7	0
Utah	0	0	0	0	0	0	0
Vermont	0	0	0	0	0	0	0
Virginia	8	811	696	87	9	17	2
Washington	0	0	0	0	0	0	0
West Virginia	1	4	4	0	0	0	0
Wisconsin	1	57	51	2	0	2	2
Wyoming	0	0	0	0	0	0	0

*Excludes American Samoa, Guam, Puerto Rico, and the Virgin Islands.
**Due to rounding, the racial/ethnic estimations sometimes add up to slightly more or less than the true total.

Table 10
TRENDS IN THE ESTIMATED NUMBER OF ENROLLMENTS
OF MINORITY STUDENTS IN BASIC RN PROGRAMS, 1991 TO 1996[1]

YEAR	BLACK		HISPANIC		ASIAN		AMERICAN INDIAN	
	Number	Percent	Number	Percent	Number	Percent	Number	Percent
ALL REPORTING RN PROGRAMS								
1991	21,529	9.1	7,349	3.1	6,947	2.9	1,700	0.7
1992	22,147	8.6	7,667	3.0	8,306	3.2	1,685	0.6
1993	23,501	8.7	8,114	3.0	8,811	3.3	1,797	0.7
1994	24,055	9.0	8,696	3.2	9,566	3.6	1,869	0.7
1995	24,621	9.4	9,039	3.5	10,444	4.0	1,900	0.7
1996	23,611	9.9	9,227	3.9	10,529	4.4	1,816	0.8
BACCALAUREATE PROGRAMS								
1991	9,239	10.2	3,066	3.4	3,063	3.4	530	0.6
1992	9,154	9.0	2,896	2.8	3,966	3.9	663	0.6
1993	10,257	9.3	3,219	2.9	4,383	4.0	614	0.5
1994	10,327	9.2	3,664	3.2	4,855	4.3	698	0.6
1995	10,884	9.9	3,647	3.3	5,635	5.1	666	0.6
1996	10,648	10.3	3,990	3.9	5,925	5.7	676	0.7
ASSOCIATE DEGREE PROGRAMS								
1991	10,577	8.5	3,861	3.1	3,391	2.7	1,115	0.9
1992	11,327	8.5	4,237	3.2	3,687	2.8	976	0.7
1993	11,710	8.5	4,405	3.2	3,818	2.8	1,132	0.8
1994	12,397	9.1	4,478	3.3	4,093	3.0	1,123	0.8
1995	12,606	9.3	4,922	3.6	4,265	3.1	1,193	0.9
1996	11,838	9.7	4,882	4.0	4,206	3.4	1,109	0.9
DIPLOMA PROGRAMS								
1991	1,710	7.5	416	1.8	493	2.2	52	0.2
1992	1,666	7.2	534	2.3	653	2.8	46	0.2
1993	1,534	6.9	490	2.2	610	2.7	51	0.2
1994	1,331	6.7	554	2.8	618	3.1	48	0.2
1995	1,131	6.9	470	2.8	544	3.3	41	0.2
1996	1,125	8.8	355	2.8	398	3.1	31	0.2

[1] Excludes American Samoa, Guam, Puerto Rico, and the Virgin Islands.

Table 11
ESTIMATED NUMBER OF STUDENT GRADUATIONS FROM ALL BASIC
RN PROGRAMS, BY RACE/ETHNICITY, NLN REGION AND STATE: 1996*

NLN REGION AND STATE	NUMBER OF PROGRAMS	TOTAL** NUMBER OF GRADUATIONS	NUMBER OF GRADUATIONS				
			White	Black	Hispanic	Asian	American Indian
United States	1,508	94,757	81,334	6,508	3,197	3,060	629
North Atlantic	327	22,371	19,040	1,995	630	617	84
Midwest	442	26,149	24,044	1,009	364	615	103
South	514	33,983	28,986	3,050	1,119	581	240
West	225	12,254	9,264	454	1,084	1,247	202
Alabama	36	2,758	2,297	408	17	25	11
Alaska	2	95	76	6	4	2	7
Arizona	17	1,057	941	14	66	25	12
Arkansas	22	1,202	1,088	86	8	9	10
California	95	5,371	3,368	344	694	886	75
Colorado	16	911	778	36	71	15	9
Connecticut	16	838	757	51	16	13	1
Delaware	7	370	331	35	1	3	0
D. of Columbia	5	328	231	59	14	23	2
Florida	39	4,182	3,366	434	253	106	24
Georgia	33	2,378	2,042	276	32	25	1
Hawaii	7	362	197	1	10	152	0
Idaho	7	296	276	3	6	8	5
Illinois	73	4,461	3,722	293	137	304	5
Indiana	46	2,682	2,506	94	41	29	12
Iowa	42	1,737	1,673	32	9	15	5
Kansas	29	1,330	1,238	46	19	17	9
Kentucky	34	1,909	1,859	28	1	9	10
Louisiana	23	1,757	1,489	215	18	24	11
Maine	15	548	537	1	3	2	3
Maryland	23	1,616	1,298	209	33	73	3
Massachusetts	44	2,742	2,505	144	44	43	5
Michigan	48	3,428	3,175	129	41	62	17
Minnesota	24	1,529	1,457	20	9	32	10
Mississippi	23	1,605	1,443	150	7	2	3
Missouri	50	2,532	2,378	94	20	34	4
Montana	5	241	206	2	13	4	16
Nebraska	14	834	777	14	17	24	3
Nevada	6	297	262	4	8	20	4
New Hampshire	9	502	494	1	2	4	1
New Jersey	37	2,246	1,765	232	110	125	16
New Mexico	15	603	430	9	122	7	36
New York	101	8,521	6,576	1,209	364	319	47
North Carolina	62	2,994	2,640	253	36	40	26
North Dakota	7	301	285	1	2	4	9
Ohio	67	4,913	4,595	198	39	64	12
Oklahoma	28	1,295	1,068	53	27	33	113
Oregon	16	797	712	6	25	33	21
Pennsylvania	82	5,599	5,224	240	61	71	5
Rhode Island	7	508	453	23	15	12	4
South Carolina	21	1,234	1,092	124	6	12	0
South Dakota	10	403	388	1	0	3	11
Tennessee	36	2,363	2,159	173	12	17	2
Texas	77	5,564	4,329	417	649	148	21
Utah	7	702	656	1	21	19	5
Vermont	4	169	167	0	0	2	0
Virginia	37	2,291	1,995	218	17	55	5
Washington	24	1,302	1,148	28	38	76	12
West Virginia	20	835	821	6	3	3	0
Wisconsin	32	1,999	1,850	87	30	27	6
Wyoming	8	220	214	0	6	0	0

*Excludes American Samoa, Guam, Puerto Rico, and the Virgin Islands.
**Due to rounding, the racial/ethnic estimations sometimes add up to slightly more or less than the true total.

61

Table 12
ESTIMATED NUMBER OF STUDENT GRADUATIONS FROM BASIC BACCALAUREATE
NURSING PROGRAMS, BY RACE/ETHNICITY, NLN REGION AND STATE: 1995–96*

NLN REGION AND STATE	NUMBER OF PROGRAMS	TOTAL** NUMBER OF GRADUATIONS	NUMBER OF GRADUATIONS				
			White	Black	Hispanic	Asian	American Indian
United States	523	32,413	27,428	2,272	1,128	1,396	176
North Atlantic	117	7,084	6,062	566	182	252	18
Midwest	164	10,123	9,179	412	167	322	38
South	181	11,239	9,217	1,173	509	276	61
West	61	3,967	2,970	121	270	546	59
Alabama	13	1,017	848	142	9	15	3
Alaska	1	71	53	6	4	2	6
Arizona	4	341	294	5	20	14	8
Arkansas	9	323	290	23	3	5	2
California	24	1,475	885	78	156	337	17
Colorado	7	439	383	12	24	13	7
Connecticut	8	378	351	14	5	8	0
Delaware	2	165	142	22	0	1	0
D. of Columbia	4	283	231	24	9	18	2
Florida	13	905	608	138	131	27	1
Georgia	14	849	728	88	15	15	1
Hawaii	3	157	67	1	1	87	0
Idaho	3	103	88	3	3	8	3
Illinois	27	1,634	1,390	77	47	118	2
Indiana	20	1,166	1,049	64	27	22	4
Iowa	12	406	388	7	4	5	1
Kansas	11	595	548	25	7	11	3
Kentucky	10	526	508	8	1	5	3
Louisiana	13	885	708	151	8	14	4
Maine	7	251	243	1	1	2	2
Maryland	7	609	496	63	13	36	1
Massachusetts	16	903	834	37	14	14	3
Michigan	15	1,153	996	76	20	51	9
Minnesota	9	540	510	6	4	16	3
Mississippi	7	522	463	54	4	0	2
Missouri	17	936	856	44	14	21	1
Montana	2	136	123	2	4	4	3
Nebraska	6	578	528	13	14	23	1
Nevada	2	111	84	2	8	15	2
New Hampshire	3	125	123	0	1	1	0
New Jersey	9	432	317	41	36	38	0
New Mexico	2	91	61	1	20	3	6
New York	33	2,096	1,562	325	84	117	4
North Carolina	12	853	722	102	7	18	5
North Dakota	7	301	285	1	2	4	9
Ohio	22	1,667	1,545	75	13	31	2
Oklahoma	11	436	346	22	10	26	30
Oregon	3	296	258	3	11	21	3
Pennsylvania	31	2,124	1,957	94	25	46	4
Rhode Island	3	266	243	8	7	5	3
South Carolina	8	437	379	49	2	7	0
South Dakota	4	199	197	0	0	1	1
Tennessee	18	906	834	57	4	10	1
Texas	25	1,984	1,421	192	297	67	7
Utah	3	248	230	1	5	11	1
Vermont	1	61	59	0	0	2	0
Virginia	12	657	543	81	4	28	1
Washington	6	443	392	7	10	31	3
West Virginia	9	330	323	3	1	3	0
Wisconsin	14	948	887	24	15	19	2
Wyoming	1	56	52	0	4	0	0

*Excludes American Samoa, Guam, Puerto Rico, and the Virgin Islands.
**Due to rounding, the racial/ethnic estimations sometimes add up to slightly more or less
  than the true total.

Table 13
ESTIMATED NUMBER OF STUDENT GRADUATIONS FROM ASSOCIATE DEGREE
NURSING PROGRAMS, BY RACE/ETHNICITY, NLN REGION AND STATE: 1995-96*

NLN REGION AND STATE	NUMBER OF PROGRAMS	TOTAL** NUMBER OF GRADUATIONS	NUMBER OF GRADUATIONS				
			White	Black	Hispanic	Asian	American Indian
United States	876	56,641	48,792	3,952	1,927	1,516	439
North Atlantic	152	12,489	10,487	1,285	373	282	61
Midwest	250	14,579	13,556	546	165	242	62
South	310	21,286	18,455	1,788	575	291	173
West	164	8,287	6,294	333	814	701	143
Alabama	23	1,741	1,449	266	8	10	8
Alaska	1	24	23	0	0	0	1
Arizona	13	716	647	9	46	11	4
Arkansas	11	622	569	42	3	3	4
California	71	3,896	2,483	266	538	549	58
Colorado	9	472	395	24	47	2	2
Connecticut	6	349	312	25	8	3	1
Delaware	4	186	170	13	1	2	0
D. of Columbia	1	45	0	35	5	5	0
Florida	26	3,277	2,758	296	122	79	23
Georgia	19	1,529	1,314	188	17	10	0
Hawaii	4	205	130	0	9	65	0
Idaho	4	193	188	0	3	0	2
Illinois	42	2,656	2,239	202	66	146	3
Indiana	25	1,453	1,398	27	14	6	8
Iowa	25	1,091	1,057	17	3	9	3
Kansas	18	735	690	21	12	6	6
Kentucky	24	1,383	1,351	20	0	4	7
Louisiana	9	827	740	63	7	10	7
Maine	8	297	294	0	2	0	1
Maryland	14	914	717	140	19	36	2
Massachusetts	21	1,415	1,276	89	26	22	2
Michigan	31	2,218	2,124	51	21	11	8
Minnesota	15	989	947	14	5	16	7
Mississippi	16	1,083	980	96	3	2	1
Missouri	30	1,343	1,278	44	6	10	3
Montana	3	105	83	0	9	0	13
Nebraska	7	199	194	1	1	1	2
Nevada	4	186	178	2	0	5	2
New Hampshire	6	377	371	1	1	3	1
New Jersey	14	1,158	959	132	29	29	11
New Mexico	13	512	369	8	102	4	30
New York	63	6,247	4,854	878	275	195	43
North Carolina	47	1,965	1,762	139	25	18	21
North Dakota	0	0	0	0	0	0	0
Ohio	34	2,688	2,521	106	22	28	8
Oklahoma	17	859	722	31	17	7	83
Oregon	13	501	454	3	14	12	18
Pennsylvania	23	2,101	1,968	98	18	16	1
Rhode Island	3	206	175	14	8	7	1
South Carolina	13	797	713	75	4	5	0
South Dakota	6	204	191	1	0	2	10
Tennessee	14	1,151	1,038	100	8	5	0
Texas	50	3,372	2,733	216	330	80	13
Utah	4	454	426	0	16	8	4
Vermont	3	108	108	0	0	0	0
Virginia	17	1,317	1,166	114	10	22	4
Washington	18	859	756	21	28	45	9
West Virginia	10	449	443	2	2	0	0
Wisconsin	17	1,003	917	62	15	7	4
Wyoming	7	164	162	0	2	0	0

*Excludes American Samoa, Guam, Puerto Rico, and the Virgin Islands.
**Due to rounding, the racial/ethnic estimations sometimes add up to slightly more or less than the true total.

Table 14
ESTIMATED NUMBER OF STUDENT GRADUATIONS FROM DIPLOMA
NURSING PROGRAMS, BY RACE/ETHNICITY, NLN REGION AND STATE: 1995-96*

NLN REGION AND STATE	NUMBER OF PROGRAMS	TOTAL** NUMBER OF GRADUATIONS	NUMBER OF GRADUATIONS				
			White	Black	Hispanic	Asian	American Indian
United States	109	5,703	5,114	284	142	148	14
North Atlantic	58	2,798	2,491	144	75	83	5
Midwest	28	1,447	1,309	51	32	51	3
South	23	1,458	1,314	89	35	14	6
West	0	0	0	0	0	0	0
Alabama	0	0	0	0	0	0	0
Alaska	0	0	0	0	0	0	0
Arizona	0	0	0	0	0	0	0
Arkansas	2	257	229	21	2	1	4
California	0	0	0	0	0	0	0
Colorado	0	0	0	0	0	0	0
Connecticut	2	111	94	12	3	2	0
Delaware	1	19	19	0	0	0	0
D. of Columbia	0	0	0	0	0	0	0
Florida	0	0	0	0	0	0	0
Georgia	0	0	0	0	0	0	0
Hawaii	0	0	0	0	0	0	0
Idaho	0	0	0	0	0	0	0
Illinois	4	171	93	14	24	40	0
Indiana	1	63	59	3	0	1	0
Iowa	5	240	228	8	2	1	1
Kansas	0	0	0	0	0	0	0
Kentucky	0	0	0	0	0	0	0
Louisiana	1	45	41	1	3	0	0
Maine	0	0	0	0	0	0	0
Maryland	2	93	85	6	1	1	0
Massachusetts	7	424	395	18	4	7	0
Michigan	2	57	55	2	0	0	0
Minnesota	0	0	0	0	0	0	0
Mississippi	0	0	0	0	0	0	0
Missouri	3	253	244	6	0	3	0
Montana	0	0	0	0	0	0	0
Nebraska	1	57	55	0	2	0	0
Nevada	0	0	0	0	0	0	0
New Hampshire	0	0	0	0	0	0	0
New Jersey	14	656	489	59	45	58	5
New Mexico	0	0	0	0	0	0	0
New York	5	178	160	6	5	7	0
North Carolina	3	176	156	12	4	4	0
North Dakota	0	0	0	0	0	0	0
Ohio	11	558	529	17	4	5	2
Oklahoma	0	0	0	0	0	0	0
Oregon	0	0	0	0	0	0	0
Pennsylvania	28	1,374	1,299	48	18	9	0
Rhode Island	1	36	35	1	0	0	0
South Carolina	0	0	0	0	0	0	0
South Dakota	0	0	0	0	0	0	0
Tennessee	4	306	287	16	0	2	1
Texas	2	208	175	9	22	1	1
Utah	0	0	0	0	0	0	0
Vermont	0	0	0	0	0	0	0
Virginia	8	317	286	23	3	5	0
Washington	0	0	0	0	0	0	0
West Virginia	1	56	55	1	0	0	0
Wisconsin	1	48	46	1	0	1	0
Wyoming	0	0	0	0	0	0	0

*Excludes American Samoa, Guam, Puerto Rico, and the Virgin Islands.
**Due to rounding, the racial/ethnic estimations sometimes add up to slightly more or less than the true total.

Table 15
TRENDS IN THE ESTIMATED NUMBER OF GRADUATIONS
OF MINORITY STUDENTS FROM BASIC RN PROGRAMS, 1990-91 TO 1995-96[1]

YEAR	BLACK		HISPANIC		ASIAN		AMERICAN INDIAN	
	Number	Percent	Number	Percent	Number	Percent	Number	Percent
ALL REPORTING RN PROGRAMS								
1990-91	5,350	7.4	2,026	2.8	1,809	2.5	363	0.5
1991-92	5,786	7.2	2,404	3.0	2,037	2.5	461	0.6
1992-93	6,024	6.8	2,340	2.6	2,270	2.6	610	0.7
1993-94	6,455	6.8	2,841	3.0	2,796	2.9	566	0.6
1994-95	6,751	7.0	3,021	3.1	2,942	3.0	622	0.6
1995-96	6,508	6.9	3,197	3.4	3,060	3.2	629	0.7
BACCALAUREATE PROGRAMS								
1990-91	1,552	8.0	525	2.7	765	4.0	115	0.6
1991-92	1,670	7.8	641	3.0	744	3.5	126	0.6
1992-93	1,799	7.4	587	2.4	918	3.8	193	0.8
1993-94	1,912	6.6	870	3.0	1,116	3.9	133	0.5
1994-95	2,277	7.3	913	2.9	1,258	4.0	170	0.5
1995-96	2,272	7.0	1,128	3.5	1,396	4.3	176	0.5
ASSOCIATE DEGREE PROGRAMS								
1990-91	3,415	7.3	1,307	2.8	937	2.0	236	0.5
1991-92	3,762	7.1	1,605	3.0	1,179	2.2	322	0.6
1992-93	3,860	6.8	1,584	2.8	1,211	2.1	405	0.7
1993-94	4,150	7.1	1,790	3.0	1,475	2.5	409	0.7
1994-95	4,085	7.0	1,917	3.3	1,519	2.6	431	0.7
1995-96	3,952	7.0	1,927	3.4	1,516	2.7	439	0.8
DIPLOMA PROGRAMS								
1990-91	381	6.2	196	3.2	109	1.8	11	0.2
1991-92	354	5.4	158	2.4	114	1.7	13	0.2
1992-93	365	5.3	169	2.4	141	2.0	12	0.2
1993-94	393	5.5	181	2.5	205	2.9	24	0.3
1994-95	389	5.5	191	2.7	165	2.3	21	0.3
1995-96	284	5.0	142	2.5	148	2.6	14	0.2

[1] Excludes American Samoa, Guam, Puerto Rico, and the Virgin Islands.

Table 16
ANNUAL ADMISSIONS OF MEN TO ALL BASIC RN PROGRAMS,
BY NLN REGION: 1995–96*

ALL REPORTING RN PROGRAMS

NLN REGION	NUMBER OF PROGRAMS REPORTING	TOTAL ENROLLMENT	MEN	
			Number	Percent
All Regions	1,162	93,484	11,735	12.5
North Atlantic	261	24,419	3,221	13.2
Midwest	318	23,831	2,539	10.7
South	422	34,301	4,400	12.8
West	161	10,933	1,575	14.4

BACCALAUREATE PROGRAMS

All Regions	395	30,633	3,810	12.4
North Atlantic	86	6,956	744	10.7
Midwest	119	9,093	1,072	11.8
South	145	10,739	1,433	13.3
West	45	3,845	561	14.6

ASSOCIATE DEGREE PROGRAMS

All Regions	674	56,958	7,238	12.7
North Atlantic	125	14,348	2,053	14.3
Midwest	177	13,365	1,332	10.0
South	256	22,157	2,839	12.8
West	116	7,088	1,014	14.3

DIPLOMA PROGRAMS

All Regions	93	5,893	687	11.7
North Atlantic	50	3,115	424	13.6
Midwest	22	1,373	135	9.8
South	21	1,405	128	9.1
West	0	0	0	0

*Excludes American Samoa, Guam, Puerto Rico, and the Virgin Islands.

Table 17
TRENDS IN ADMISSIONS OF MEN
TO ALL BASIC RN PROGRAMS: 1986–1996[1]

YEAR	NUMBER OF PROGRAMS REPORTING	MEN	
		Number	Percent
ALL REPORTING RN PROGRAMS			
1986	1,228	5,715	6.6
1987	1,192	5,302	7.2
1988	1,257	5,958	7.3
1989	1,272	7,558	8.2
1991	1,194	10,033	10.7
1992	1,219	12,568	12.0
1993	1,243	14,111	12.9
1994	1,205	14,463	13.5
1995	1,206	13,947	13.3
1996	1,162	11,735	12.5
BACCALAUREATE PROGRAMS			
1986	382	1,783	6.0
1987	370	1,560	7.1
1988	412	1,675	6.7
1989	429	1,820	7.0
1991	412	3,003	10.4
1992	405	3,837	12.2
1993	412	4,434	12.6
1994	399	4,369	12.4
1995	404	4,486	12.8
1996	395	3,810	12.4
ASSOCIATE DEGREE PROGRAMS			
1986	643	3,432	7.1
1987	630	3,290	7.6
1988	682	3,726	7.6
1989	695	4,857	8.6
1991	654	6,089	10.9
1992	691	7,580	12.0
1993	711	8,357	13.1
1994	694	8,971	14.1
1995	697	8,564	13.7
1996	674	7,238	12.7
DIPLOMA PROGRAMS			
1986	203	498	5.3
1987	192	452	5.9
1988	163	557	6.8
1989	148	881	9.2
1991	128	941	10.1
1992	123	1,151	11.5
1993	120	1,320	13.6
1994	112	1,123	13.8
1995	105	897	13.0
1996	93	687	11.7

[1] Excludes American Samoa, Guam, Puerto Rico, and the Virgin Islands.

Table 18
ENROLLMENTS OF MEN TO ALL BASIC RN PROGRAMS, BY NLN REGION: 1996*

ALL REPORTING RN PROGRAMS

NLN REGION	NUMBER OF PROGRAMS REPORTING	TOTAL ENROLLMENTS	MEN Number	MEN Percent
All Regions	1,191	196,651	23,789	12.1
North Atlantic	270	54,399	6,817	12.5
Midwest	327	48,989	4,874	9.9
South	430	71,229	9,036	12.7
West	164	22,034	3,062	13.9

BACCALAUREATE PROGRAMS

All Regions	415	86,146	10,263	11.9
North Atlantic	93	20,823	2,084	10.0
Midwest	126	25,270	2,612	10.3
South	147	30,234	4,242	14.0
West	49	9,819	1,325	13.5

ASSOCIATE DEGREE PROGRAMS

All Regions	674	98,545	12,144	12.3
North Atlantic	123	27,386	3,871	14.1
Midwest	176	20,822	2,002	9.6
South	260	38,122	4,534	11.9
West	115	12,215	1,737	14.2

DIPLOMA PROGRAMS

All Regions	102	11,960	1,382	11.5
North Atlantic	54	6,190	862	13.9
Midwest	25	2,897	260	9.0
South	23	2,873	260	9.0
West	0	0	0	0

*Excludes American Samoa, Guam, Puerto Rico, and the Virgin Islands.

Table 19
TRENDS IN ENROLLMENTS OF MEN IN ALL BASIC RN PROGRAMS: 1986–1996[1]

YEAR	NUMBER OF PROGRAMS REPORTING	MEN Number	MEN Percent
ALL REPORTING RN PROGRAMS			
1986	1,228	8,259	4.4
1988	1,257	10,100	6.2
1989	1,272	12,404	6.9
1991	1,194	19,072	9.9
1992	1,157	22,823	11.1
1993	1,289	30,005	12.4
1994	1,236	28,875	12.6
1995	1,240	29,061	13.1
1996	1,191	23,789	12.1
BACCALAUREATE PROGRAMS			
1986	382	2,219	2.4
1988	412	3,363	5.4
1989	429	3,867	5.9
1991	412	6,973	9.8
1992	370	8,353	11.0
1993	438	12,470	12.3
1994	418	11,717	12.0
1995	421	11,330	12.1
1996	415	10,263	11.9
ASSOCIATE DEGREE PROGRAMS			
1986	643	4,992	6.7
1988	682	5,539	6.8
1989	695	7,033	7.5
1991	654	10,068	10.1
1992	669	12,178	11.2
1993	730	14,924	12.6
1994	700	14,705	13.2
1995	705	15,841	14.0
1996	674	12,144	12.3
DIPLOMA PROGRAMS			
1986	203	1,048	4.9
1988	163	1,198	6.5
1989	148	1,504	7.8
1991	128	2,031	9.6
1992	118	2,292	10.8
1993	121	2,611	12.2
1994	118	2,453	12.9
1995	114	1,890	12.1
1996	102	1,382	11.5

[1] Excludes American Samoa, Guam, Puerto Rico, and the Virgin Islands.

Table 20
GRADUATIONS OF MEN FROM ALL BASIC RN PROGRAMS, BY NLN REGION: 1995–96[1]

ALL REPORTING RN PROGRAMS

NLN REGION	NUMBER OF PROGRAMS REPORTING	TOTAL GRADUATIONS	MEN Number	MEN Percent
All Regions	1,156	75,721	9,478	12.5
North Atlantic	264	18,522	2,384	12.9
Midwest	314	19,685	2,034	10.3
South	415	28,058	3,740	13.3
West	163	9,456	1,320	14.0

BACCALAUREATE PROGRAMS

NLN REGION	NUMBER OF PROGRAMS REPORTING	TOTAL GRADUATIONS	MEN Number	MEN Percent
All Regions	391	26,457	3,326	12.6
North Atlantic	89	5,810	657	11.3
Midwest	120	8,337	928	11.1
South	137	9,025	1,334	14.8
West	45	3,285	407	12.4

ASSOCIATE DEGREE PROGRAMS

NLN REGION	NUMBER OF PROGRAMS REPORTING	TOTAL GRADUATIONS	MEN Number	MEN Percent
All Regions	667	43,986	5,521	12.5
North Atlantic	121	10,107	1,389	13.7
Midwest	171	10,081	977	9.7
South	257	17,627	2,242	12.7
West	118	6,171	913	14.8

DIPLOMA PROGRAMS

NLN REGION	NUMBER OF PROGRAMS REPORTING	TOTAL GRADUATIONS	MEN Number	MEN Percent
All Regions	98	5,278	631	11.9
North Atlantic	54	2,605	338	13.0
Midwest	23	1,267	129	10.2
South	21	1,406	164	11.7
West	0	0	0	0

[1]Excludes American Samoa, Guam, Puerto Rico, and the Virgin Islands.

Table 21
TRENDS IN GRADUATIONS OF MEN FROM ALL BASIC RN PROGRAMS: 1986–1996[1]

YEAR	NUMBER OF PROGRAMS REPORTING	MEN Number	MEN Percent
ALL REPORTING RN PROGRAMS			
1986	1,228	3,916	5.5
1988	1,237	3,264	5.7
1989	1,272	3,080	5.7
1991	1,194	4,745	8.4
1992	1,006	6,178	9.9
1993	1,167	7,808	10.5
1994	1,178	9,130	11.4
1995	1,171	10,140	12.4
1996	1,156	9,478	12.5
BACCALAUREATE PROGRAMS			
1986	382	1,146	4.3
1988	393	983	5.2
1989	429	851	5.0
1991	412	1,201	8.2
1992	298	1,639	10.4
1993	376	2,233	10.5
1994	393	2,816	11.1
1995	390	3,290	12.2
1996	391	3,326	12.6
ASSOCIATE DEGREE PROGRAMS			
1986	643	2,326	6.8
1988	681	1,896	5.9
1989	695	1,989	6.0
1991	654	3,106	8.5
1992	609	4,027	9.7
1993	679	4,897	10.4
1994	672	5,509	11.5
1995	672	5,991	12.4
1996	667	5,521	12.5
DIPLOMA PROGRAMS			
1986	203	444	4.4
1988	163	385	6.7
1989	148	240	5.2
1991	128	438	8.0
1992	99	512	9.7
1993	112	678	10.6
1994	113	805	12.0
1995	109	859	13.0
1996	98	631	11.9

[1] Excludes American Samoa, Guam, Puerto Rico, and the Virgin Islands.